How Children Grieve

How Children Grieve

CORINNE MASUR

ROBINSON

ROBINSON

First published in the United States of America in 2024 by Alcove Press,
an imprint of The Quick Brown Fox & Company LLC.

First published in Great Britain in 2024 by Robinson

1 3 5 7 9 10 8 6 4 2

A CIP catalogue record for this book
is available from the British Library.

ISBN: 978-1-47214-954-1

Printed and bound in Great Britain by
Clays Ltd, Elcograf S.p.A.

Papers used by Robinson are from well-managed forests
and other responsible sources.

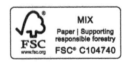

Robinson
An imprint of
Little, Brown Book Group
Carmelite House
50 Victoria Embankment
London EC4Y 0DZ

An Hachette UK Company
www.hachette.co.uk

www.littlebrown.co.uk

For all of those dear to me who have died during my lifetime:
my parents, Jack and Barbara; my aunts Ida, May, Annabelle,
and Lillian; my uncles Lou, Fred, and David;
and my friends Sue and Carol. You have taught me what my
grief looks and feels like.

CONTENTS

Contents

Part 2
Helping the Grieving Child

PREFACE

"Give sorrow words: the grief that does not speak whispers the o'erwrought heart and bids it break."
　　　　　　　　　—*Macbeth*, William Shakespeare[1]

When I was fourteen, my father died.

He was in his bedroom, taking a nap before a dinner party he and my mother were hosting. And then, just after he got up from his bed, he had a massive heart attack.

My mother found him when she went up to change for the party. She didn't call 911. She didn't scream or cry. She just said, "Something's happened to Daddy." Hearing this, my sister ran out the back door to get our next-door neighbor, who was a doctor.

Dr. Marbury immediately came over, sped up the stairs to my parents' bedroom, and then came down again several minutes later.

I overheard him say to my mother, "I'm sorry, Barbara, there's nothing I can do."

I sat on a chair in the dining room as the coroner came, as dessert burned in the oven, and as the guests rang the doorbell. My mother answered the door, still wearing her apron from cooking, and I heard her friends' voices go from hearty hellos to hushed whispers of "Oh, I'm so sorry."

Too shocked to do anything else, they all came in. At some point, a well-meaning woman came into the dining room where I sat and asked if I would like to go be with my mother. I didn't answer her—and I didn't move.

Following the realization that my father had died, I became immobile. I was quite literally in the "freeze" part of the "fight-flight-freeze" response to danger. Few if any thoughts crossed my mind. I just sat in the chair, staring straight ahead. I was experiencing traumatic shock, something I could not have named or explained at the time.

Not all fourteen-year-olds would have responded this way. Some would have screamed and cried, some would have run to the bedroom to try to help their father, some would have clung to their mother or their sister. But I reacted by freezing.

Hours later I must have gone up to my room because I remember waking up in my bed the next morning feeling fine.

And then I remembered that my father had died.

From that day on, my life, my family, and my identity were irrevocably changed. Time was divided into "before" and "after."

I was now the girl whose father had died, the girl who no one knew what to say to, the girl who did not know what to say to herself.

In some ways, I went on autopilot. I returned to school on Monday, and when a kind teacher asked if I wanted to take the test scheduled for that day, I just said yes, because I didn't know what else to do. I went on with my day, acting as though I were the same person I had been on the Friday before. I could do all the things I always did, but—even though I did not want to acknowledge it—life would never be the same, and I would never be the same.

When I went outside after school to the pickup line of cars, my mother was not there. Instead, I saw my brother standing beside his little red car. My brother was supposed to be away at medical school. My brother never picked me up from school. And that brought it all back again.

In my family, we did not talk about our feelings. I didn't know that my mother was so distraught that she wasn't able to drive to pick me up. In fact, I had no idea how she was feeling.

And no one asked how I was doing. Nor did I ask anyone how they were doing. We went through the motions—the funeral, which was so awful, with everyone looking at us, the awkward condolence calls, the giving away of my father's clothes, the dividing up of the jobs my father did around the house. But we didn't really talk about any of it.

I had no idea how to mourn a father.

I kept my thoughts and feelings to myself. I tried to be of help to my mother, to keep her company, to pay her the compliments my father might once have given, but neither she nor I really knew what we were doing.

And the sad fact is that I stayed on autopilot for a long time.

I had no idea how to talk about my father. Growing up in a family where feelings were not openly acknowledged or shared, I hadn't a clue how to start.

My grief never really had a chance.

In some way, I stayed frozen in that chair in the dining room for years, unable to feel much or even to know what I should be feeling. But as time went by, the experience of my father's sudden death, and my complete cluelessness about how to feel and how to behave afterward turned to curiosity.

How did other people grieve? How did other families handle loss? This curiosity is why I took up the subject of grief and loss when it came time to choose a specialty in psychology.

Like many children and teenagers, I needed help to know how to express my grief. I needed help in exploring the feelings I had, and I needed explicit encouragement to do so. While I was not conscious of doing this at the time, rather than feeling and expressing my complete disbelief, my sadness, and my confusion, I just developed a way to handle life. I became extremely self-sufficient and kept literally *all* of my thoughts and feelings about my father's death inside. I even managed to keep some of these thoughts and feelings so well hidden that I didn't know about them myself.

But there is danger in unexpressed grief.

The feelings that are not acknowledged or shared can turn into bodily or psychological symptoms. Sometimes a bereaved child will experience strange aches and pains, or they may feel persistently sad. They may withdraw and find it hard to connect with friends and family or to allow themselves to put energy into new relationships.

On the other hand, some children or teenagers will rush to form new attachments to fill the void left by the lost loved one and to distract themselves from the mourning they need to do.

I did some of each of these. And none of these "solutions" were particularly beneficial to me nor are they beneficial to any child's development.

Children and teens need support and modeling for their grief. Without such help, some children are unable to recognize their own feelings or to value them sufficiently to devote the energy to exploring them and expressing them. When feelings are kept inside, grief and mourning are truncated, and sometimes they are stalled or go awry, falling into the territory of symptom formation and/or prolonged, persistent, or pathological grief reactions.

My mother knew none of this. She did not know what I was feeling. She did not know what would be helpful to me. She did not understand that I needed help with my grief, or, for that matter, that she needed help with her own grief. In truth, she was as frozen as I was. We both needed a better model for grieving. We both needed help expressing our shock and sadness and feelings of complete helplessness.

As a teenager, I did not know how to actively grieve—I just tried to survive.

For my doctoral dissertation, I chose to write about childhood bereavement. In learning about loss in childhood, I learned about myself and what it was that happened to me emotionally and psychologically when my father died. As they say, much of research is actually "MEsearch."

Later, as a child psychologist and psychoanalyst, I used what I learned, both academically and personally, in my effort to help children and teenagers—and their parents—to do things differently than I had—that is, to learn to recognize their own feelings and to express them.

Then I began to write some more: first a book for mental health professionals on loss in childhood, When a Child Grieves: Psychoanalytic Understanding and Technique, and now, this book—which I am writing for parents, teachers, grandparents, aunts, uncles, clergy, coaches—anyone who wants to help children or teenagers to mourn, to move forward, and to make meaning of terrible loss, without having to keep all the feelings inside.

Because all children, regardless of their age or the type of loss they have suffered, require love, support, guidance, and understanding to scaffold and assist them as they learn to navigate their way through the pain.

All children need someone to answer their questions and support their feelings in order to prevent them from keeping their grief frozen inside them.

All children need the adults around them to be willing to try to understand their loss from their point of view. This kind of support helps children to avoid the pitfalls of a pathological grief reaction— that is, experiencing frozen, delayed, or prolonged grief and/or developing bodily symptoms to indirectly express their grief.

All caregivers of grieving children (mainly parents or guardians, but also engaged teachers, clergy, or other mentors) need help in understanding what children and teens may feel when they are grieving. All need help learning how to listen to these children and teens. This is especially true for caregivers who are grieving the same loss as the child they are caring for.

Ultimately, when a child's grief is understood from their point of view as well as in the context of their developmental stage, the resulting support can be both encompassing and profound.

In this book, I give the guidance adults need to learn how to help a grieving child. I explore how grief affects children at each age and stage of development. I discuss the many types of grief, including the death of different family members. I also look at the manner of loss, including a special kind of loss called ambiguous loss, as well as loss

that comes not from death but from a dramatic change in life circumstance or environment.

   All of this will be helpful to you in understanding the impact of
loss on children and in deepening your awareness of the way grief is
experienced and processed by the children in your life.

   I look forward, in the coming pages, to helping you understand
the experience of loss for the children you love.

What Adults Miss

Behind childhood grief is a world of feelings and beliefs, shaped and colored by the individual child's age, personality, family circumstances, culture, and stage of development.

Adults who try to help a grieving child, lacking direct access to the child's inner world, often look at the child's behavior and form ideas of what the child is feeling and how they are affected based on external impressions.

And in doing so, they can miss a *lot*.

They can miss what the child feels about the loss, they can miss what the child understands about the loss, they can miss the child's misconceptions about death and loss in general. They can miss the child's fantasies about this loss in particular and what role the child believes she played in causing the loss to happen.

There is a lot that is important *not* to miss.

When a child loses someone they love, the child doesn't stop loving that person. The child may not even really believe that person is gone. The child may start searching for them everywhere they go, and each night they may see their lost loved one in their dreams.

Children don't stop needing the people they lose, and they don't stop wanting them. Children continue to yearn for them, not just for the care they provided or the fun they had together, but for *them*— their presence, their companionship, their love.

But when a child loses a beloved person, their love for that person becomes a one-sided equation. It is an unreciprocated, lonely kind of love that involves powerful feelings of missing their lost loved one.

All this missing can feel different for each child. It can feel like pain. Or it can feel like confusion. It can feel like an ongoing emptiness. It can feel like an ache in the pit of the stomach or a headache that never ends. Some children stop eating. Some start eating too much to fill that emptiness.

Most children can't bear the feeling for long, and they take breaks from it by returning to play and school activities. This could make it seem like the child is no longer grieving. But, in fact, it does not mean the pain, the emptiness, the yearning, or most of all, the loving has stopped.

For example, when Chloe was four years old, her grandmother died. She had been close to her grandmother, seeing her at least once almost every week of her life. After being told that her grandmother had died, Chloe went off to the family room. Her parents observed her playing quietly with her dolls, and they were relieved. They felt that she had taken the news very well and saw her as returning to her normal activities.

Several weeks later, when Chloe began to have trouble at bedtime, refusing to go to sleep without one parent or the other lying down with her, they did not link this to her experience of her grandmother's death. They felt that she was being "clingy" without good reason.

The truth was that Chloe was very frightened. She had been told that her Nana had "gone to sleep forever and was now with God in Heaven," so she was afraid to go to sleep, fearing that she would never wake up.

When Chloe went to play with her dolls after being told the news of her grandmother's death, she had played a game of putting her dolls to bed and having them go to sleep and then to Heaven. She played this over and over, trying to work out both how someone could sleep forever and where Heaven was. In addition to becoming frightened to go to sleep, Chloe was feeling more fearful of separations in general. She also had powerful feelings of missing her Nana and didn't understand why she couldn't still go to her house to visit.

Chloe's parents had not thought to wonder how Chloe would understand the words they said to her about her grandmother's death. They had four children altogether, and Chloe was the third. They were happy with Chloe's adaptation to the news of her grandmother's death and very caught up with their own grief, the reactions of their other three children and the funeral arrangements.

Chloe's story is just one example of how children might react to loss.

In *How Children Grieve*, I take an in-depth look at the internal world of the child in order to help caregivers better understand the nuances of feeling and fantasy a child may experience when confronted by loss. I discuss how unique each child's understanding and reaction to loss are and how strongly they are shaped by her personality, family circumstance, age, stage of development, and culture. I talk about losses of all kinds, including losses due to death, abandonment, deployment, divorce, and immigration. And I talk about how some less obvious kinds of loss can be something hardly noticed by the family, known as ambiguous loss. Other losses, of course, can take the form of a sudden and major trauma, obvious to all.

The loss of a loved one, in particular, is devastating for anyone, but our hearts break especially for children because losing a beloved person is so painful and potentially damaging for them.

So when considering our children's psychological health it is important *not* to miss their feelings and inner experiences when confronted by loss. We need to understand—from their perspectives— what loss feels like, how they may react to it, and how they may be affected by it.

It is important to remember that loss in childhood is not just something to get over; it affects the child for years to come. It changes how they feel, who they are, and how they see and experience the world. Whatever kind of loss a child suffers needs to be processed and metabolized over time. And children need help with this.

There are many ways that a child can react to loss and be affected by it. A major loss in childhood can serve as an impediment to development, it can be managed and coped with, or it can even provide motivation for growth.

I have divided the book into two main parts. First, in part 1, I consider loss and grief from infancy to adolescence. I explore what grief is and how it affects children. I consider the way grief is experienced and processed at the different stages of development. Finally, in this first part I explore the different kinds of losses children experience, from the death of a parent, sibling, or grandparent to a beloved caregiver or friend, as well as the manner of loss, be it sudden, violent, or ambiguous.

So with an understanding of grief and how it affects children at different stages of development, the reader can then move on to the second part of the book, which focuses on helping the grieving child.

First, I consider the grief of the adult caregiver, discussing the difficulties of suffering grief while also caring for a grieving child. I emphasize the importance of the caregiver receiving adequate support, so they are then able to provide the essential care to the grieving child in their life needs.

Then I discuss how to help children experiencing each of the many forms of loss in childhood.

I will refer to experts in the field of loss, to the research in this area, and to literature, as well as offering some individual examples from my clinical work, and my own personal experience, in order to bring to life the child's experience of loss.

The subject of loss is particularly pertinent at this moment in history as we recover from a major pandemic, as we live through several major wars, and as we experience natural disasters, climate change, and ever-escalating gun violence.

These events are dramatically increasing the number of children who are experiencing losses. The wars around the world, including in Russia and Ukraine and in Israel and Gaza, Yemen, Sudan, Afghanistan, Ethiopia, Syria, Libya, Central African Republic, Congo,

Myanmar and Mali have already taken tens of thousands of lives. Of those who have died, many were parents, leaving orphaned or partially orphaned children behind. And during the coronavirus pandemic, an extremely large number of children suffered the loss of parents and other loved ones. Shockingly, more than 10.5 million children lost one or both parents or caregivers due to Covid-19 according to data released in September 2022. At least 5.2 million children suffered the loss of a caretaker in the first twenty months of the pandemic alone, and in the United States, by March 2022, over 200,000 children had lost a primary or secondary caregiver due to Covid. In fact, so far, one in four Covid deaths represents the loss of a parent or primary caregiver for at least one child.[1]

Southeast Asia and Africa suffered the greatest rate of losses, with one out of every fifty children affected compared with one out of one hundred fifty children in the Americas, according to a research letter published in *JAMA Pediatrics*.[2]

These circumstances have brought all sorts of loss for children in addition to the losses they have suffered due to death. During the pandemic most children suffered fear of disease. As a result, many children the world over lost their sense of safety and security. During the pandemic many children also lost some degree of contact with friends and extended family for weeks and months at a time. All lost in-person classroom time. Even worse, over the past few years many children had to leave their schools, homes, and even their countries whether due to war, food scarcity, economic or political hardship, or violence.

Even in normal times, without a pandemic or a war, children suffer multiple kinds of loss that we often do not even acknowledge. When a parent becomes depressed, this is a loss for a child. When a parent goes on a long trip for business or is deployed by the military, this is a loss. When a parent goes back to work after having worked at home or after having been a stay-at-home parent, this is a loss. When a sibling moves away from home, this is a loss. And when a beloved babysitter stops working for a family, this is a loss. When a best friend switches schools, this is a loss. And when a family moves to a new city, state, or country, this is a loss that contains multiple losses within it.

For many children, the experience of these losses has been further exacerbated by the difficulties in accessing the love and support needed to help them through such difficult times. Whether due to Covid, war, natural disaster, or any other tragedy, parents, grandparents, teachers, and adults in general may all have been less available than usual over the past several years. These adults may also have been preoccupied and worried themselves.

It is also important for us, as adults, to remember that our job is to help children learn about the possibility of loss—including death—before they experience loss and to help them with their losses when they do occur. It is our job to aid the children we love to express their feelings, to listen to what these children have to say about their feelings, to understand with them what their losses mean to them, and to work on understanding these losses from their perspective. This is crucial because children can feel very alone when they have lost someone or something dear to them. They need a great deal of support and accompaniment through loss. Without support, without warmth and caring, and without answers to their many questions, children may become blind to their own real feelings. They may misunderstand their own role in the loss in a way that undermines their self-concept and self-confidence. They may develop pathological variants of the grief process. And without adequate understanding and help, they may become adults who are not able to be sensitive to their own feelings or the feelings and needs of others—including their own children—when they experience loss.

So, loss in childhood comes with risks. Compared to nonbereaved children, bereaved children are at higher risk for a range of mental and behavioral health problems, including depression, posttraumatic stress reactions, substance use,[3] decreased academic performance,[4] and suicide.[5]

Of those children and teens who experience the loss of a close loved one, 10 to 18 percent will go on to develop Persistent Complex Bereavement Disorder, a relatively new diagnosis to be included in the *Diagnostic and Statistical Manual of Mental Disorders* and one that involves numerous debilitating symptoms and a great deal of distress for bereaved children and teens.[6]

We are talking about a lot of children who are grieving. And in the United States, we are talking about these children living in the context of a society that tends to avoid discussion of death and grief and which maintains the belief that it is important to protect children from the knowledge of death.

But this is a kind of wishful thinking. By as early as three years of age, children are aware of death, whether we talk with them about it or not. They have seen dead bugs and dead animals by the side of the road. They have heard about killings and deaths in their families, in their neighborhoods, or on the news, whether on TV or on social media, as well as in movies and video games.

If we do not talk to children about what they see and hear about death, if we do not explain to them what it's all about, these children will be unprepared for experiencing their own losses. They will have no idea how to understand death and how to express their feelings about death and loss. And if we are not talking about these subjects with them, they may feel they are not supposed to talk about them either.

In this country, death is often siloed. We think that we protect our children by not discussing it or by keeping them from going to the funerals of relatives. But what we are really doing is leaving children all alone with the thoughts and feelings they are already having.

Following a loss, when we do speak with children about death, when we do help them to understand what has happened, and when we do help them with their feelings, many can experience growth from loss. Children can find great meaning in their losses; they can grow in sensitivity and depth, and they can become more empathic to the painful experiences of others.

While you might be familiar with the "stages of grief," I won't be including them as a framework in this book. These stages have been attributed to Elisabeth Kübler-Ross, an eminent death researcher and psychiatrist. But the truth is that she did not see these stages in people who had experienced loss. She observed and categorized these stages during her research on dying patients. Only years after her original work on death and dying did she and David Kessler adapt them to those who were mourning,[7] and there has been a great deal of controversy regarding whether these stages actually occur in those who are grieving.

In fact, recent research has shown that the idea that there are stages people must go through and tasks they must accomplish to complete the mourning process may not be true at all. George Bonanno, a professor of psychology at Columbia University and one of the most noted researchers on grief and mourning, says that much of what we have believed about what is necessary to grieve is simply untrue and not documented by research. According to Bonanno, people follow different patterns and different trajectories for grief across time. This is true for children as well, and this is the position I take throughout the book.

Crucially, *How Children Grieve* provides a basis for understanding the experience and the needs of individual children who have experienced loss. The information presented here is based on sound developmental theory rather than opinion. Following graduate training in clinical psychology, postgraduate training in child and adult psychoanalysis, and over forty years of experience working with grieving children, I have found that the best way to understand children's feelings and needs is based on both a highly individualistic and a developmental approach. That is, we understand the child as a unique individual with particular perceptions and understandings all her own, and we also understand her based on her age, stage of development, existing personality, family circumstance, culture, and the type of loss she has suffered.

Grief may look a little bit different for every child, but by learning what is typical of children at each age, by listening and observing closely, you will have the tools you need to support the children in your life on their grief journeys.

As you dive into the book, feel free to read it as presented or use the table of contents to jump directly to a chapter that particularly addresses your situation. You may also want to take some notes in a journal or on your phone to remind you of what you need to do to help the child in your life.

At the end of the book, I've included a brief "How to Help the Grieving Child" checklist (page 261). Once you've read the book, you can refer back to this checklist to help you remember the key things that will be most helpful to you.

Throughout the book, I include many case examples. To protect the confidentiality of those I see in my clinical practice, the cases presented are either heavily disguised or they are conglomerates of real people. Only with express permission do I use real patient material and when I do, I always use pseudonyms rather than the real names of the people involved.

I would also like to add that I use the terms "parent," "mother," and "primary caretaker" interchangeably as not all children are cared for exclusively by their parents and not all parents who care for children are mothers.

Finally, I also use "her" or "they" when talking about the children who have suffered loss—in part to correct a historical imbalance. Traditionally, the subjects of discussion in books and elsewhere have been referred to as "he." It is time that we also use "she" and "they." In this book, when I say "she/her" or "they/them" I am referring to all children and teens—including those who identify as male, female, nonbinary, transgender, queer, or other.

PART 1

Loss and Grief from Infancy to Adolescence

Depending on a child's age and stage of development, she will understand loss differently, perceive loss differently, feel differently about loss, and be affected by loss differently. In this section, I will define grief and mourning, and then I will explain in very specific terms how children of different ages and at different stages respond to loss.

CHAPTER 1

What Are Grief and Mourning, and How Do They Affect Children?

I define grief quite simply as what one feels following a loss. Grief can feel crushingly sad, or it can feel like numbness. It can come in waves, or it can wait a month and then mow you down. It can take forms that do not feel—or look—at all like sadness.

Grief is personal. It is unique to each grieving person. It may be private, or it may be loud and public.

There is no right way and no wrong way to grieve or mourn.

And this is true for children as well as adults.

When children run around and play following a loss, people will say that the children are not grieving—or that they are not grieving appropriately.

This is simply untrue. Children grieve in their own ways.

For children as well as for adults, every loss is unique and every loss is experienced uniquely.

After years of studying bereavement, one of researcher George Bonanno's most consistent findings is that "bereavement is not a one-dimensional experience. It's not the same for everyone and there do not appear to be specific stages that everyone must go through."[1]

Mourning, on the other hand, is often defined as our outward expression of loss. But here I will talk about it as the internal process of grieving a loss.

This process takes time. It requires energy and focus. It involves a reworking of the relationship with the person who has died so that it transforms from an external, real-world relationship to an internal one. And in this process, parts of the lost loved one can become part of the mourner.

And how do we know when mourning is moving forward?

When mourning is successful, the bereaved person is able to move ahead in life and to make room for new relationships.

Writers and clinicians have tried to tame the process of mourning by categorizing it in various ways. But in the end, mourning can take any number of shapes. As I mentioned, there is no set of stages everyone must pass through. It is just like other painful, out of control experiences in our lives: it is messy and there is no road map.

And for mourning to occur, the first thing that must happen is that there must be an acknowledgement that a loss has occurred.

This may seem obvious. But when you lose someone you really love, it is sometimes hard to accept that they are really gone. And this is doubly true for children because, especially before the age of five, children do not understand what death is. They do not understand that it is permanent. They do not realize that someone who dies cannot and will not come back.

Being unable to acknowledge that a loved one is really gone can be part of what makes mourning difficult for children, especially young children.

Children under the age of five do not fully understand the concept of death without a great deal of help from adults.

When someone dies, young children often expect them to come back, they may wish them to come back, and they may believe that they will come back. As a result, without help from adults, they may not feel all the sad feelings that come with understanding that someone is truly lost.

Even children over five, who may understand the concept of the permanence of death a little better, need help remembering that when someone has died, they cannot come back and they will not come back no matter what we wish for. Additionally, while children who are six and seven and eight may understand that death is permanent, they often think that if someone leaves or dies it must either be their fault or someone else's fault.

At each age, there are developmental differences that caregivers must understand and consider in order to truly understand and help the child with their grief and mourning.

Without adults to remind the child, misunderstandings can stay in their mind. The child may think that if only she is good enough, the person she lost will come back. Or she may think that if only she had been good enough in the first place, they would never have gone away.

If the child does not truly understand that a person or a thing they lost is really gone permanently, they may not feel as sad as they would have if they did understand that the person is gone forever— and thus, mourning cannot really occur, or it may be delayed until they fully understand and accept what has happened.

For similar reasons, it can also be hard for children to mourn other kinds of losses such as parental separation, deployment to the military, the loss of a home to a natural disaster, or when friends or relatives move away. In these cases, where the person could possibly come back or when the child thinks that the home and possessions might possibly be restored, it is hard for the child to know what to feel. If a child does not know if her parents will get back together, if her deployed parent will come back, or if her uncle who was lost in the flood might be found, it is very hard to know whether to feel sad and whether to mourn. The child is left in a kind of limbo. This is called ambiguous loss, and I will discuss this at length in chapter 5.

It is more straightforward for a child when someone or something is gone and cannot come back due to death. But in both loss due to death and in ambiguous loss, there can be mourning—and for mourning to occur the child must experience the loss, acknowledge the loss, and have internal reactions to and feelings about the loss.

So, how does mourning start?

Initially, the mourner may feel shocked.

It may take a few days, a few weeks, or even a few months to fully acknowledge what has happened and for feelings to set in.

Then there can be a period of intense pain—crying and yearning and wishing for the person to come back. These feelings often come in waves, and they may show up at unexpected moments—often when the child sees something or does something that the person who is gone might have seen or done with them.

After a period of time the child can generally begin to think about and remember who or what has been lost without as much shock or pain as they felt initially, to sort out what they miss and what part of the lost person or thing they want to hold on to, and meaning can be made of the loss; it can be processed and understood. After this has happened, the sad feelings generally diminish—and while they may not go away entirely, they are usually far less painful than they were in the beginning. The enormous sadness can be replaced by occasional memories that evoke shorter periods of sad feelings.

Throughout this process, the shape of each child's grief is determined by their age, their stage of development, their relationship with the person (or thing) they lost, and their own particular personality and life circumstances. No two children experience loss in exactly the same way—even if they have lost the same thing. To one child, the loss of a father when they are twelve may feel catastrophic and result in a long-lasting depression. For another child, the loss of a father at twelve may feel freeing and promote independence—after their initial shock and sadness have diminished.

Some children bounce back more quickly than others. There is an increasing amount of research being done on what has been called resilience—the idea that some infants, children, and adults weather adverse events more easily than others and some children raised under adverse conditions do better than others. But the answers to the question of what makes one individual more resilient than another are very complicated and not fully understood. At present, we believe that resilience is probably rooted in a person's neurobiology, culture, family, society, socioeconomic status, and individual personality.

So, let's think about resilience. One might think that if an infant is robust and healthy and has a laid-back temperament, then it is likely that she will weather changes in her life better than an infant who is highly reactive, more sensitive, or more fragile. As it turns out, this is not always true. In a study of Masai children affected by severe drought, it turned out the more difficult, fussy children fared better than the more laid-back children.[2] Perhaps it is the feistier children, the ones who register discomfort and make vigorous demands on their parents to provide comfort, who actually withstand adversity better.

Also, the adequacy of the person who takes care of the child after the adverse event is important. The more sensitive the caretaker is to the moods, feelings, and needs of the infant or child (and, if it is the primary caretaker who has been lost, the more they can replicate the caretaking patterns of the caretaker who left if these were positive patterns), the more likely it is that the infant or child will recover from adversity and adapt more quickly.

Of course the socioeconomic status of the family will also influence how a child will respond to adversity such as loss. Families with more resources, including good housing, good schools, and access to good medical and psychological services will be able to provide a more stable and supportive system within which the child can recover. However, this is not to say that a child from a well-resourced family will not suffer terribly from the loss of a parent nor that a child from a community with fewer resources will not find love and support and the help they need from within their family and community. This is merely a generalization.

So what does determine whether a child does better or worse when exposed to a difficult event such as a loss?

Ann Masten, an authority on the subject, describes a variety of factors that I have adapted to the subject of loss:

- **Dose.** The severity (or dose) of the loss will, in part, determine a child's reaction. So, of course, the loss of a distant relative will likely be less difficult for a child than the loss of a beloved parent. And multiple losses at once will be much more difficult to recover from than a single loss.
- **Timing.** A child will be more vulnerable to suffering greater effects from loss during certain developmental periods than others. For example, the loss of a parent during the first three years of life will be quite devastating to a child, while the loss of a parent later in adolescence will be very difficult in many ways, but perhaps not as damaging as a similar loss at a much earlier age.
- **Close attachments.** Having close attachments has been shown over and over to be an extremely protective factor in helping a child to be less drastically affected by loss and more likely to recover more fully. Having loving family and friends with whom the grieving child has strong relationships supports the child during the grieving process, supplies the love she needs, and sustains her throughout the rest of her life.
- **Intelligence and executive functioning.** More intelligent children who are more capable of keeping themselves organized have been shown to do better under adverse conditions.
- **Cultural belief systems and rituals.** Having a belief system and/or a set of routines and rituals around loss, whether religious or cultural, has been found to be protective in helping children respond with more resilience to loss.[3]

In this chapter, I will explain how key factors such as culture, personality, and loneliness affect the shape of a child's grief, and how understanding these factors can aid you to truly help children who are grieving. Later, in the sections on each age and stage of development, I will explain further about the timing and dose of loss.

How Culture Shapes the Child's Reaction to Loss

In many cultures there are customs, traditions, and expectations for the way that children should feel and behave following the loss of a loved one. Some of these are explicit (spoken and known) and some are implicit (unspoken and often less well acknowledged) but still expected. In other cultures and traditions there is an absence of ritual or routine.

For example, among North American atheists, death may be talked about very little, and there may be few, if any, formal rituals around the death of a family member. In my own family, there were no set rituals at all. When a beloved uncle of mine died, there was no funeral, no burial service, just a cocktail party, which took place months after he died. Although he would have loved the cocktail party—especially the snacks—it was not necessarily helpful for many of the members of my family. There was very little in the way of overt mourning. There was really no structure to scaffold the grieving of the children—or the adults. If we wanted to say goodbye, we each had to figure out how to do so on our own.

Similarly, when my father died, there was a funeral, but that was all—no prescribed period of mourning, no rules or customs in place to help us decide when to go back to work or school, and no lighting of candles or religious ceremonies to ritualize the remembering of my father in the years after his death.

So, the culture within which I lived provided little in the way of rituals or routines for mourning. For any child experiencing a loss, the scaffolding—or the lack thereof—provided by their family and larger culture within which they live will affect the child's experience of loss as well as her mourning process.

To use another example, in his memoir, *Did Ye Hear Mammy Died?*, Séamas O'Reilly, whose mother died when he was five, describes his family's approach to grief. He says they didn't want to suffer the pity of outsiders or cause any "fuss," since fuss of any kind "is like kryptonite to Northern Irish people."[4]

He goes on to say that it was odd for him to realize, as an adult, how much of his homeland he had internalized, even at the age of five, and how many of the unspoken assumptions, behaviors, and rhythms of thought had become his own.

He realized that, as a little boy, he had been living by the platitudes he had been brought up with: "'Don't make a fuss,' 'it's no big deal' and 'ah sure lookit the horse has bolted what good will whining do?'"[5] All of these kept him from expressing his shock and grief when his mother died.

A child brought up in Northern Ireland, or a child of parents brought up there who have emigrated to another country, may be prone to keeping their most difficult feelings to themselves—as might the children of other cultures where the expression of feelings is not encouraged.

However, in some cultures, grief and mourning may be more openly expressed. The children's film *Coco* shows that in certain cultures in Mexico, grief, mourning, and celebration of the dead are parts of life, especially on the Day of the Dead, which is celebrated every year.

But it is not only the general culture of the family's community, whether religious or ethnic, but also each family's particular interpretation of that culture that will influence how the family and the children contained within it mourn.

Within a given culture, individual families have their own way of doing things, which may not align exactly with the culture they are part of. Their own customs are superimposed over the customs of their forebears and their community so that a given religious or cultural background may not determine the unique way that a particular family deals with feelings—including grief and mourning.

In my practice, I have seen children and adolescents from varying backgrounds and cultures. In each and every case, there were aspects of grief and mourning that were well supported by the particular family and culture from which the child came, and there were also elements of the child's experience that the family completely missed and which they had to be helped to understand.

For example, one little girl's grandmother died in the village from which her father came in Africa. The family went back to the village and joined a large community of mourners. When the little girl, who was eight at the time, came back from the trip, she told me that she felt so loved while she was in her grandmother's village. She experienced the attention of her cousins and great-aunts and uncles as very supportive and helpful to her as she watched her father mourn the loss of his mother.

At the same time, when she came back to her family's apartment in the United States and went back to school with her friends, she felt strange. Her family did not continue to carry out any of the customs or rituals she had been a part of in her grandmother's village. She wasn't sure what to do to show her sympathy for her father now that the family was back to its normal routine. She missed the relatives she had met and been surrounded by in Africa. And she also felt somehow different from her friends here in the United States and unsure how to be with them.

It was important for me to help this child figure out how to talk to her father. She needed to tell him how strange it felt to be back home and how she couldn't really understand how to integrate the experience she had had in Africa with her life here.

Her father was very moved by his daughter's confusion, and he agreed to take her to some of the community events attended by people from his parents' village who had immigrated to Philadelphia. He also found a couple of ways to memorialize his mother at home that were in keeping with some of the traditional rituals. He had not realized that connection to his culture might be important to his daughter and that she might need help to understand how she could be both an American girl and a girl with roots and relatives in another country.

Later, this little girl told me about some of the new friends she had made at the gatherings her father took her to and how knowing them helped her to feel more connected to her grandmother and the life her grandmother had lived.

Another family I worked with was Ukrainian and Jewish. The parents had come to the United States separately and met here. Neither was observant when it came to their religion, but they both valued their religious and their national identities.

When the children were nine and thirteen, their father was killed in a car accident. The mother came to me as soon as she was released from the hospital (having been in the car with her husband and having sustained injuries of her own). She wanted help with what to tell her children.

She did not have religious beliefs within which to frame or explain death to the children nor did she have religious rituals to help her and her children to formally say goodbye to their father and husband. She felt lost and unsure about how to proceed.

Some Jewish families who are more observant in their religious practice have prescribed prayers to say, ways to memorialize their loved one, and certain ways to explain death and loss to children. They may wear black, they may rip their clothes or wear a ripped ribbon symbolic of ripped clothing, and they may stay home to receive visitors for a period called shiva, in which a short service is held every night for seven days, and friends and family members drop by. But this mother and her children did not have these customs to follow.

What they did have, however, were grandparents from both sides of the family—and in what may have been a different, sort of less specific expression of both religious tradition and cultural practice, both couples were immediately available in all ways to this woman and her two children. Lovingly, they alternated weeks, sleeping over at the family's house and helping the children to feel cared for.

Neither religion nor culture are necessarily a sure framework for families when loss occurs. But each affects how a family experiences and deals with death and loss, as does the lack of religion or strong cultural affiliation.

How Personality Shapes the Experience of Loss and How Loss Shapes Personality

The experience of loss and the degree to which an individual is affected by loss are also influenced by their preexisting personality.

Whether a child is particularly sensitive or whether she is especially resilient, whether she is outgoing or more introverted, whether she is easily able to ask for help or whether she tries to cope on her own will all affect the way that she responds to loss.

Fascinating information on the way that this occurs in adults was obtained by a group of researchers, led by Dr. Geddam Subhasree, who performed a study on 237 people who had lost a close loved one to Covid. These researchers wanted to understand the role of personality in the outcome of mourning.

Interestingly, they found that people who have a sense of being able to affect others and their environment (called self-efficacy) are more likely to return to normal functioning after a significant loss. The team summarized the findings of their study saying that a high degree of self-efficacy served as a protective factor against depression and grief among the bereaved individuals who lost their loved ones due to Covid.[6]

In their review of the professional literature on this subject, Subhasree and colleagues also found that individuals who were characterized as having what is called openness, who have a tendency to accept new experiences, who feel less nervous through disappointments, and who believe in themselves, also fare far better following loss. Similarly, individuals who are agreeable, those with conscientiousness traits, those who exercise their abilities and recognize their limitations, and those who set realistic goals all tend to have increased ability to persevere and persist in challenging situations.

While this study did not include children and adolescents, I think we can generalize from their findings and hypothesize that children who have some of the characteristics listed above will generally recover more easily from loss.

I suspect that children who have a high degree of self-efficacy—that is, children who can take action in their lives, who feel they can affect the opinions of the adults around them, and who feel they can solve problems for themselves—are more likely to do better after a loss.

Similarly, children who are open to new experiences, who can adapt to change better, and who can accept new circumstances will also do better when confronted by loss.

Like the adults in the study, children who believe in themselves, who trust that they can withstand difficult things, and who are less nervous when met with disappointment are likely to do better when they lose a loved one.

Finally, children who are conscientious, agreeable, and able to persist under difficult circumstances, like the adults in the study, are also likely to do better following loss than children who do not have these characteristics.

As for the effect of loss on the development of personality? Well, loss shapes different people differently, but it will definitely affect the development of the personality of the infant, child, or teen who experiences the loss.

In my family, my father's death affected each of the four of us in a dramatic way, but it did not affect each of us in the same way.

For example, one of my sisters may or may not have been my father's favorite (we debate this to this day). But she did spend a great deal of time with him, and she loved him and depended on him in many ways. My father and this sister shared a stamp collection and spent hours together on Sundays putting their stamps into albums. When this sister needed a summer job, he found her one through a professional connection. And when she wanted advice on a variety of matters, she went to him.

My father died when my sister was in her second year of college, and life was never the same for her. The person she loved most and depended on for help when she needed it was suddenly gone. Her expectations for his involvement in her life going forward collapsed. My father would not be at her college graduation, and he would not see her go on to graduate school or to receive her Ph.D. He would not be available for any love or help or advice at all. And for the most part, she had put all her eggs in one basket—our father.

My sister became depressed—and this was a depression that plagued her for years. She was deeply sad and alone. She suffered. She looked to my mother for some of the interest and support my father had shown her, but she was disappointed over and over again. After some years, she began to turn to our older brother for some of the advice and help that she had once sought from my father. She had depended on my father, and going forward, she depended on our brother as well as on other friends and family.

I was different.

First of all, I was fourteen when my father died as opposed to her twenty. Second, I had a different personality makeup than she. When my father died, I became less dependent, and I did not try to find others on whom to depend. I sought out opportunities to do things on my own. When I was sixteen, I decided to get an after-school job, and when I was seventeen, I chose to attend an unconventional college far from home, and unlike any that the others in my family had attended.

I was not my father's favorite, my grades were not as good as my sister's, and I had given up, long before he died, on being able to please him. So my sister and I were very different in this respect.

At the same time, I was uncomfortable feeling helpless. So, over time, I figured out how to keep my own counsel and make my own decisions. Doing this allowed me to avoid feeling too vulnerable or too sad. If I could rely on myself, I did not have to feel helpless, and I did not have to miss my father too much.

After my father's death, my sister's dependence continued in some ways, while my independence blossomed.

So, my father's death affected my sister and her life trajectory in certain ways, while it affected me and my personality development in other ways. She suffered, felt quite alone, and transferred her dependence on my father elsewhere. Meanwhile, I turned to myself, hoping, and often believing, that I could handle things myself.

This is just one example of the different ways that loss can affect two different children—in this case, even within the same family.

And, as you can see from the experience I had following my father's death, personality growth can occur as a result of loss. This is not what people generally think about when they consider the effects of early loss on children and teens—and yet it is real.

For years, two researchers, Lawrence Calhoun and Richard Tedeschi, studied the positive effects of trauma—including loss. Contrary to public opinion, they found that individuals who had suffered significant trauma often experienced positive changes. These changes include improved relationships, new possibilities for life, a greater appreciation for life, a greater sense of personal strength, and increased spiritual development.

They also found some interesting contradictions. People they interviewed said things like "I am more vulnerable, yet stronger." Individuals who experienced traumatic events tended to talk about their increased sense of vulnerability; however, these same people also reported an increased sense of their own capacities to survive and prevail.

Another experience often reported by trauma survivors was a need to talk with other people about the traumatic events, which tended to deepen some of their personal relationships. Some also found themselves becoming more comfortable with intimacy and having a greater sense of compassion for others who experienced life difficulties.[7]

In my practice, a teenager whose father had died at the beginning of Covid said to me, "My dad's death gave me a different perspective. I used to think that if a friendship ended or someone died, all the time you put into that relationship was wasted. Now I think that it was valuable. I would rather have had my dad for the time I had him rather than some other dad who was around longer."

This young woman gained a new perspective and came to a new appreciation of the relationships in her life. She came to understand the importance of the person that her father was despite her lifelong frustration with having had an older dad. And she also recognized that relationships are important in their own right, even if they end prematurely.

Calhoun and Tedeschi also found that people who faced trauma were more likely to become engaged with fundamental existential questions about death and the purpose of life. A commonly reported change was for the individual to value the smaller things in life more and to also consider the religious, spiritual, and existential components of life. A common theme for many people in this study was that after a traumatic event philosophies of life can became more fully developed, satisfying, and meaningful.[8]

Researchers such as Calhoun and Tedeschi have found that growth can occur not despite adversity but because of it.

It is true that they looked predominantly at adults, but interestingly, very similar findings have been found in research on bereaved children.

In a study of what helps and hinders children and adolescents who lose a parent, Jessica Koblenz found multiple areas of growth in many of the children she interviewed.[9]

Seventy-three percent of the participants in her study felt that navigating and understanding death at an early age made them grow up faster.

Some said they responded to loss by embracing life. One said, "I have a heightened sense of life, not wasting time, and not having regrets." According to some grief theorists, this renewed sense of life is an adaptive form of meaning-making following loss.

Many of the children Koblenz interviewed said that support helped them to get through their loss. This finding is important because traditional psychological and psychiatric views of bereavement have minimized the role of relationships and support from others in coping with loss. However, more recently, evidence has shown that relational support plays a crucial role in a child's ability to cope after a loss and may actually improve and intensify some existing relationships.

Interestingly, participants in Koblenz's study stated that their most helpful source of support were other mourning children who could relate with their exact position.

Koblenz also found that becoming self-reliant was a coping strategy that some of the participants in her study utilized. (This sounded very familiar to me!) In her study, kids said that they began to rely more on themselves once they decided that they could no longer depend on others. For some, it was easier to express they "were strong" and "could handle it alone" than to acknowledge their loneliness.

Koblenz says that the sentiment of "needing to be strong" was expressed by many participants and reflected their inability to convey vulnerability. As one participant said of her childhood loss, "Everyone always said, 'You're so strong.' No one ever said, 'It's okay if you're not.'" From this Koblenz concluded that applauding children's ability to handle their grief alone may make it difficult for them to feel they can be completely open and show their vulnerable selves. But some participants were able to find a balance of healthy independence while still reaching out to others in times when they needed help.

So, in sum, it can be said that personality definitely affects how one child handles loss as compared to another child. And loss definitely affects children's personality development. Some resilient children will move through their grief and go forward in their development, changed but still moving forward. Some will actually grow from loss, and other, less resilient children, will experience an interruption in forward development and will need help to move forward. You can read more about growth from loss in chapter 11 (page 240).

The Loneliness of Loss

As Helen Macdonald said in her memoir *H Is for Hawk*, "Bereavement . . . It happens to everyone. But you feel it alone."[10]

And this can be especially true for children and teenagers.

For example, a young woman I interviewed said, "What makes me feel most lonely ever since my mom died [is that] consciously or unconsciously, I've been searching for maternal figures at school and at college. It becomes another sad thing, [like] 'this lady is lovely; I wish she could be like my mom but she can't.' . . . Even with my stepmom, she's sort of maternal, but there's a distance; you miss your mom for your mom as a person but also for a mom."

Children and teens may feel very lonely after a major loss. Often they will not have any friends who have experienced what they have. Or if they do, they may feel reluctant to talk about their experience. And to rid themselves of their loneliness, they may wish to replace their lost loved one right away. Or they may want to shut themselves off from needing anyone.

Children and teens who are feeling very lonely and sad may feel ashamed of their feelings, imagining that others have not felt as they do. Or they may feel that they don't know how to put what they are feeling into words.

They may feel they don't even know what they feel.

When I was at my lowest moments in my first year of college, I would go outside and look at the sky, feeling terribly alone and missing my father. This had absolutely nothing to do with the reality of whether my father could have actually helped me to feel better had he still been alive. I gazed at the sky more out of my feelings of sheer aloneness. And one thing that came to mind when I felt this way was the fact that my father was gone.

On one particular occasion during freshman year, as I thought of my father, I looked at the night sky and talked to him. I asked him why he had left me. And, for one of the first times since his death, I really cried.

But I did not talk to any of the real, living people around me about this. I wasn't accustomed to talking to others about my deepest feelings.

This is not an unusual experience for children and teens. Many do not have the first clue about how to approach a friend to reveal something personal or to ask for help. Some don't know where to begin, and others may feel they don't even deserve help.

Children and teens who have lost someone dear to them miss that person and grieve for them at all sorts of moments. Feelings of grief and sadness may take children and teenagers by surprise, welling up at the most unexpected of times. They go somewhere that they used to go with their lost loved one and they remember them. Or they need help with some homework that the person who died would have helped with and suddenly they feel bereft. Sometimes they even feel like giving up. What's the point of doing homework if their loved one isn't there?

Being unable to put the missing feelings into words, being shy about doing so, being reluctant to ask for help—or even to admit to needing help—leads to many lonely moments. And sometimes children are irritable at these times—or they may feel sleepy and go off to take a nap—when what they are actually feeling is pain.

Of course, it is essential for children to have loving family and friends who are available to notice—and to draw them out when they find it hard to talk. But it is also the case that many times missing feelings happen in private.

When a parent, friend, or close grandparent is gone, it is common for children to retreat to their rooms. It is also common for them to imagine that if only that person were present they would feel less alone and that person would be able to help or to make things better. And these feelings can occur in even the youngest of children.

Donald W. Winnicott, a British child psychoanalyst and author of innumerable books, wrote about such a child in his book *The Piggle*. He described how a little girl became very frightened at night after her mother left to go to the hospital to have a second child. The girl, who was not even two at the time, imagined her mother coming to her in the night looking dark and scary. The little girl had night terrors and nightmares for the time that her mother was gone and for several months afterward.[11]

Undoubtedly, this eighteen-month-old missed her mother terribly during her two-week absence. And what the Piggle did was quite clever, although it scared her: she brought her mother back every night with her nightmares. Evidently, having a scary mommy with her at night was better than no mommy with her at all.

This little girl was painfully aware of her mother's absence. Imagining her mother coming to her at night was the way that her young mind coped with her mother being gone.

Loneliness combined with grief is just extremely hard to bear for children of any age. Recently a young man in my practice told me exactly this. He was back from his first year of college, and he was talking about how lonely he had been at times over the course of the year. This caused him to then think about what had happened when his grandfather died several years before. He said, "When my grandfather died, my father went to comfort his mother. I wanted to talk to someone about my grandfather, but when I went into my brother's room he was under the covers—like in a tent under his sheets—so I didn't even try. He was so depressed. And then my mother was going through it too. She loved my grandfather more than she loved her own father, so she wasn't very good about it. She didn't talk to us. So I called my father, and he said he was busy and couldn't talk to me. So later my brother came downstairs and he was playing the guitar, and he hadn't been doing anything like that for the last few days, so I came down to sit in the living room with him and all of a sudden I couldn't breathe. I'd never had a panic attack before, but I was having one. My mother came in and said, 'What's wrong?' None of us were talking to each other, and it was just a big mess."

In this family, each person was suffering separately, and each in their own way. They were all grieving, but they were doing so alone.

Loneliness is a painful part of grief, but it is also a natural one. We all feel alone at times, and the loss of a loved one brings this to our consciousness. It is not necessarily a negative, however. Even children need to learn how to tolerate occasional lonely feelings, and we can help them to do this by talking about it with them and sharing stories about our own lonely moments.

So, I have said a great deal in this chapter that will be important to remember going forward. I have defined grief as what a child or teen feels following a loss. I have defined mourning as the process a child or teen goes through internally as they learn to manage their loss. How each is experienced is affected by the child's preexisting personality, and each affects how a child's personality develops going forward. Other factors that affect the degree to which a child is impacted by loss, grief, and mourning include dose, timing, the availability of others to whom the child is attached to help, the intelligence and executive functioning skills of the child, and the culture and belief system and rituals of the child's family and community. Finally, I emphasized that grief and mourning can be lonely, but they can also promote growth on the child's or teen's part. In the following chapter, I will detail how children and teens understand and experience loss at each age and stage of development. This information is crucial for caregivers and others as children at different ages understand and are affected by loss and death so differently.

CHAPTER 2

Grief at Different Ages and Stages

At fourteen, I was clearly able to understand what my neighbor meant when he said to my mother, "I'm sorry, there's nothing I can do." I understood that my father had died. I understood what death was.

But at fourteen, how would my father's death affect me? How would I grieve? And what were the implications for my future development—and for me as an adult?

And for that matter, how would my father's death have affected me had I been younger? Or older, as my brother and two sisters were?

I had no idea about these things.

In this chapter, we will look at how loss affects children, starting in earliest infancy and continuing through adolescence. Some of what you read here will surprise you, and some will seem like common sense. But all of the information will help you to understand why the children in your care who have experienced loss are behaving and thinking in the ways that they are.

The Newborn (Zero to Four Months)

Sally was just hours old when her mother was taken to the ICU due to complications from her delivery. Sally was well taken care of by the nurses in the infant nursery at the hospital, but after several days, they wondered why no one had come to visit Sally.

As it turned out, Sally's mother was a single woman who did not have a partner. She was estranged from her own family, and it did not appear that she had friends in the area.

Sally stayed in the infant nursery for three weeks while her mother slowly improved in the ICU. However, due to the severity of her mother's condition, Sally could not visit with her mother or even be held by her mother. It was not until her fourth week of life, when her mother was moved to a step-down unit, that Sally got to be held by her mother and to stay in her mother's room.

Sally had lost her mother for the first month of her life.

In utero, Sally had been familiar with her mother's bodily rhythms and with the sound of her voice, and no doubt these provided an atmosphere of safety and calm. But once she was born, Sally no longer experienced these rhythms or sounds. She was subjected to all new stimuli. Her life was made up of an ever-changing rotation of young nurses and the bright lights and hustle and bustle of the newborn nursery.

This was a difficult situation. Sally was experiencing all new sights and sounds. She did not have the familiarity of her mother's body, her mother's voice, or her mother's smell to comfort her. The nurses coddled Sally and even brought in cute outfits bought with their own money—but none of these nurses was Sally's mother. They did not have the same rhythms, their voices were different from Sally's mother, their smells were different from Sally's mother, and the environment of the newborn nursery was not in any way like her months inside her mother.

While in the nursery, Sally was fussy and hard to soothe. She seemed uncomfortable, and she did not gain weight as quickly as the doctors would have liked.

While people—including doctors—may not consider the possibility of loss affecting a newborn or young infant, it is likely that a loss like Sally's does indeed affect the early experience of the infant.

Donald Winnicott, the British child psychoanalyst referred to in chapter 1, once wrote, "There is no such thing as a baby."[1] What he meant was that a baby does not exist outside of the relationship with her mother or primary caretaker. The baby must have this relationship in order to thrive.

The death or departure of a primary caretaker represents both the loss of a critical relationship and the loss of an enormous number of interactions that help the baby regulate herself and learn how to interact with other human beings. Loss of the mother early in life is, quite simply, an enormous tragedy that deprives the young infant of so much that she needs to develop well.

Research shows that from the earliest weeks of life, loss of or separation from the primary caretaker can affect the infant's attachment style, her investment in herself, her sense of bodily and emotional safety, and many other important abilities.[2]

When I talk about loss here, I am referring both to the literal loss of the parent due to illness, departure, or death and also to other kinds of loss. When a new mother suffers a postpartum depression, or the mother of an older infant suffers any major mental illness such as severe anxiety, major depression, a manic episode, or psychosis, the infant in essence "loses" the mother and her mothering abilities (to a greater or lesser extent).

It is difficult to think about this. We do not want to imagine the pain and discomfort a young infant can experience from the loss of a parent. We may prefer to believe that they are not affected by the negative things that happen to them when they are so small.

Even in medical circles the possibility of emotional or physical pain in infancy was denied for many years. Up until the 1980s it was thought that young infants and toddlers would neither remember nor be affected by the pain they felt during medical interventions, and babies were routinely subjected to medical procedures, including surgery, without anesthesia.

A study performed in 1992, cited by Susan Coates, provided evidence to the contrary. Researchers found that the use of anesthesia vastly improved survival rates in young infants. Of those infants studied, none of the infants who were given deep anesthesia for a surgical procedure died, while nearly one-third of infants who did not receive deep anesthesia did die. It was hypothesized that the experience of pain dramatically raised the stress levels of the infants. And the stress levels of the infants directly affected whether they survived their surgeries.[3]

Like the denial of physiological pain in infancy, up until the 1970s it was also believed that infants and preadolescent children did not experience psychic pain, including the pain caused by separation from their parents.

During much of the twentieth century, parents of infants and children who were hospitalized were not allowed to visit. The need for parental love and care was considered unimportant to physical health, and separation from parents was not considered traumatic in many medical circles. The attachment needs of young children and the benefits of love and nurturing from familiar loved ones to the recovery process went completely unrecognized.

For many years it was accepted that infants did not remember what happened to them before approximately eighteen months. However, in the last several decades it has been found that the ability to form all sorts of memories may be available from the beginning of life.

In one of many such observations made by experienced psychotherapists, Susan Coates[4] reported the case of a young man who felt pain in his heels whenever he was stressed. His early history revealed he had been subjected to repeated blood tests as a newborn with the blood being taken from the heels of his feet. One explanation for the pain he felt as an adult when he was experiencing stress was that he had a bodily memory of the early pain he suffered in infancy. While anecdotal, this example is one of many that provide some evidence that very early trauma can be represented on the bodily level.

Now, how about loss? Does an infant experience sadness or pain when a parent or other close relative dies or leaves her? Was Sally's fussiness in the newborn nursery indicative of her reaction to the loss of the familiar feelings, rhythms, and sounds provided by her mother? And if so, will this event affect her at later stages of development?

Let's start with the loss of a parent. Sally's story is a real-life example of this type of loss.

Since the 1970s, research has found that newborns, starting on the first day of life, recognize their mother's voice, scent, and even her face. Many experiments have shown that the baby much prefers looking at her mother's face over looking at the faces of other people.[5] It has also been shown that newborns who are crying can be calmed by the presentation of a piece of clothing that has their mother's scent.

So we know that the newborn not only recognizes her mother visually, and prefers to look at her over others, but she is also comforted by evidence of her mother's presence or proximity through olfactory cues or smells.

According to Marshall Klauss and John Kennel,[6] who did some of the original research on infant-parent bonding, there is also evidence that the newborn who has sustained contact with her parent during the first forty-eight hours of life establishes a special and unique relationship with that parent. The baby who has had the benefit of this sustained contact in the first hours of life feels a sense of familiarity and perhaps even comfort when held by her parent, which feels very different from the experience of being cared for by an unfamiliar person.

Even more interesting is the fact that researchers have found that within the first few hours and days of life, the mother and infant set up patterns of interaction that contribute to the infant's feeling of being sensed and known by the mother.[7]

These findings suggest, by inference, that because the infant knows and feels most comfortable with her primary caretaker and feels sensed and known by them, their loss will result in discomfort, a subjective feeling of things being different and a feeling of not being intimately known, in addition to representing a potential threat to survival.

In other words, the baby becomes attached to the mother in utero and in the first days and weeks of life.

John Bowlby, a noted British researcher, psychoanalyst, and author of a three-volume series on attachment, separation, and loss, described this process. He drew from research on animal behavior when trying to understand human infants and pointed out that, like other mammals, the early attachment of the infant to the primary caretaker improves the likelihood of survival. When the baby cries, the mother feels the urgency of the cry and comes immediately, thereby ensuring the infant's safety and the provision for the baby's needs.[8]

The infant needs the mother to survive. It is evolutionarily adaptive for the very youngest of infants to recognize and to be bonded with their own mothers.

From these descriptions, we can understand that the early bonding process is bidirectional, going from mother to infant and infant to mother. The loss of either partner in the first few months of life represents an enormous disruption for the other—and in the case of the infant, interferes in the possibility for survival, both physiological and psychological.

Many studies have looked at the importance of the primary caretaker and the effect of disruptions in care on the baby. Observations and research performed by Harry Bakwin, John Bowlby, James and Joyce Robertson, Renee Spitz, and Harry Harlow in the 1940s, 1950s, and 1960s found that loss of the mother in the early months of life constitutes a significant disruption in the infant's experience and well-being. These researchers found that such a disruption could result in regression in development and difficulty in maintaining physiological and emotional regulation for the baby. They stated that if an infant was cared for by an unfamiliar adult after having formed a bond with the parent, the infant could develop a variety of physiological symptoms, including digestive difficulties, changes in elimination habits, difficulty sleeping, fussiness, and difficulty being comforted. These symptoms clearly indicate the infant's discomfort and difficulty with separation and loss of the parent.

Even before most of these studies were performed, Harry Bakwin, a pediatrician, recognized the extreme importance of the loss of the mother for young infants. In the 1930s, Bakwin noticed that there was an alarmingly high death rate of small children in New York's Bellevue Hospital. In fact, 30 to 35 percent of all infants admitted to the hospital died.

At first, doctors thought that the high death rate was due to malnutrition, to the infection for which the infants were hospitalized, or to a newly acquired infection. So, to remedy this, Bellevue Hospital replaced open wards, where infants and children occupied beds placed next to one another in long rows, with small rooms in which "masked, hooded and scrubbed nurses and physicians move[d] about cautiously so as to not stir up bacteria."[9]

The infants and children were also given high-calorie diets. Surprising the staff, these measures had no effect on the death rates of these infants and children. Bakwin noted that, despite their high-calorie diets, the babies and children did not gain weight—at least, not until after they returned home. He concluded that the total lack of mothering at the hospital and the sterile environment in the wards were damaging. As a result, hospital policy changed and nurses were encouraged to mother and cuddle the babies and children, to pick them up and play with them, and parents were invited to visit.

The results of this change in policy were dramatic. Despite the increased possibility of infection with more handling and more visitors, the death rate for infants under one year of age at Bellevue fell sharply to less than 10 percent!

Bakwin wrote a paper on these findings, which was noticed by experts all over the world.[10] Among those who were influenced by this experience was Donald Winnicott, who went on to advocate for the importance of retaining family integrity even under dangerous conditions. Winnicott went so far as to recommend keeping children with their mothers under wartime conditions such as the bombing of

London, and he wrote a letter to the World Health Organization during World War II stating just this.[11] Later studies, after the war, proved his point, demonstrating that infants and children who were sent to live in the countryside outside of London during the Blitz fared worse psychologically than those who stayed with their mothers, despite the frightening conditions.[12]

Outside of wartime, similar findings were made. At the time that Bakwin made his observations in the United States, psychiatrist Harry Edelston conducted a similar study on separation anxiety in young children in Britain, studying children who had experienced multiple admissions to the hospital without the parents being allowed to visit. He noted that these children seemed very anxious and showed disturbed behavior. According to Edelston, the "separation from home form[ed] the essentially traumatic element in the experience" and "the younger and more helpless the child the greater the separation anxiety." In all, "the determining factor seem[ed] to be the degree of rejection or insecurity felt by the child."[13]

Several years later, in 1945, Rene Spitz investigated the experience of children in orphanages and foundling hospitals in Romania, South America, and elsewhere. He observed that many of the originally normal infants in these institutions were not meeting developmental expectations and concluded that the loss of the mother—or primary caregiver—during the children's first year produced irreparable damage. Alarmingly, he observed a precipitous decline in intelligence one year after the three-month-old infants were abandoned by their mothers.[14]

Spitz captured the experiences of the infants in a black-and-white documentary called *Grief: A Peril in Infancy* (1947). In a second film, *Psychogenic Disease in Infancy* (1952), he showed the effects of emotional and maternal deprivation on the capacity for attachment in the infants.

Much more recently, starting at the end of the twentieth century, researchers have looked at the neurobiology of attachment and have found corroborating evidence for Rene Spitz's early work. Myron Hofer and his team at Columbia University[15] have found that newborn mammals suffer physiological dysregulation, disruptions in sleep-wake cycles, activity level, and sucking patterns when they experience the loss of closeness, feeding, and warmth provided by the mother. Hofer describes the importance of the relationship with the mother in the early months of life, saying that the mother provides crucial physiological regulatory functions or "hidden regulators" for the infant.

When infants are deprived of contact with their primary caregiver, when they are deprived of the love and care and familiar feelings associated with their primary caretaker, and when they are deprived of all the regulatory functions of their caretaker, the consequences can be dire. It has been found that infants who are separated from their mothers for prolonged periods (and who do not have a loving caretaker substituted for her in short order) experience an alteration in brain development and attachment behavior. For example, Romanian orphans reared in extreme physical and social isolation were found to have smaller brains, and adopted orphans from Romania and China were found to have larger amygdalae, the area of the brain associated with emotion and fear, than their nonadopted counterparts.[16]

Ultimately, an infant will not remember loss early in life in the same way that an adult remembers events that have happened to her, but that does not mean that loss will not affect the infant. The infant may have primitive memories, especially bodily memories, of disruption and discomfort. If adequate care is not provided following the separation, if the infant is put into an institutional setting or if she receives only minimal care given by unfamiliar adults who perform only the tasks necessary for her survival, there will likely be negative effects on neurological, psychological, and emotional development.

Other factors will affect the experience of loss in early infancy. These include the infant's personality and genetic makeup as well as external factors such as the adequacy of the caretaker who takes over in the absence of the mother or primary caretaker, the socioeconomic status of the family, and the culture within which the family exists.

In sum, separation from a beloved caretaker is the most profound kind of loss in infancy. Whether the caretaker has become ill, has gone away, or has died, it is all the same to the baby—the familiar patterns and rhythms of comfort are gone. The particular ways of relating that were characteristic of that loved one are now replaced by less familiar forms of relating. This is a major disruption for an infant, and it may affect her future ability to trust and to relate as well as potentially affecting her ability to self-regulate and to have a solid sense of self.

As the baby grows older, separation and loss will be felt and experienced in other ways.

Older Infants (Four Months to One Year)

When Gerald was eight months old, his mother, Lucy, who was Gerald's sole caretaker, became acutely depressed. She stayed in bed each day and could not care for Gerald. Gerald's grandmother came to stay with them while his mother was so depressed, and although his grandmother was very familiar with his routines and his likes and dislikes, she found that he was very fussy and seemed dissatisfied with anything she did. He cried when he saw her. He cried and cried when she fed him, and he fussed for over an hour at nap time and each night when she tried to put him to sleep.

He had previously been a baby who was fairly easy to please. He had always been alert and interested in what was going on around him, and he had begun to crawl and to enjoy exploring all over his house, including places he was told repeatedly not to go.

But after his mother started to become depressed, Gerald became less active himself. He seemed to go backward in development, preferring to sit on the floor close to his mother's legs while she sat on the couch.

By the time Gerald's grandmother came to stay, Gerald seemed less good-natured. He looked pale, and he was less interested in playing and less curious than he had been.

After her mother arrived and insisted that she get help, Gerald's mother began to receive treatment for her depression. Over the next several weeks she improved to the point that she could get out of bed and begin to again take care of Gerald. Gradually, she started to initiate the games and routines she and Gerald had enjoyed together before she became so depressed. Gerald initially seemed standoffish with his mother—arching away when she first started to hold him again and refusing the spoon when she tried to feed him. But gradually Gerald resumed his previously good relationship with his mother and welcomed her caretaking.

Between four and eight months, there is a real bond between the infant and the mother or the primary caretaker. The baby of several months loves and is attached to her parents and caretakers and they fulfill a huge number of important roles for her. These include not just daily care but also the provision of love, nurturing, soothing, and opportunities for reciprocal communication, intellectual and emotional stimulation, and play. The parent or primary caretaker does so much each and every day that facilitates the baby's development and provides help with bodily and emotional regulation. They mirror the baby's feelings, providing emotional feedback in reaction to the baby's behaviors. They respond to and provide social cues, they soothe the baby when she is upset, and they help her to relax when she needs to sleep.

Also, from between four and eight months, the infant begins to understand that the parent or caretaker and she are separate. Prior to this time, she is less aware of the difference between her own feelings and needs and those of her caretaker. Starting around six to eight months of age, she may be more distressed than previously when she realizes her caregiver or parent is out of sight, and she may feel more helpless and alone when this happens. This can be especially acute after she begins to crawl and she is able to get further away from her caretaker under her own steam.

She may also become upset when people other than one of her parents or familiar caretakers try to hold her. This is what is often called "stranger anxiety." But in fact, it is the baby's recognition that she is with someone who is *not* her mother or other very familiar person. She is very aware of the difference between her familiar caretakers and others, and she does not like to be far from them or to feel that they are far from her. Over time, trust is built when the caretaker returns again and again after each absence.

At this age, the baby's relationship with others also expands. Siblings, grandparents, friends, and a nanny or babysitter who spend a great deal of time with the baby become much more important to her. They may provide joy and be a source of comfort. For example, a seven-month-old may already delight in watching her siblings or she may have a particular smile for grandpa or be especially comforted by grandma's holding and soothing.

So, a baby of four to eight months will be highly distressed if a parent or other beloved caretaker leaves and does not come back. She may cry when her mother walks out of the room and she may scream to get her to come back or attempt to crawl after her. If her mother does not return or if the baby cannot find her mother, this will be very upsetting.

The baby at this age wants to be in proximity to her much loved caretaker. She does not yet understand the difference between a temporary departure and a permanent disappearance.

When Gerald's mother was suddenly less available emotionally, he was distressed. Even though he knew his grandmother and was generally comfortable in her arms, he was upset by the prolonged emotional absence of his most beloved and most familiar caretaker, his mother.

Of course, an infant cannot understand what it means for someone to get sick, to become depressed, or to die, but they do register the absence of someone they love and they do feel distress and discomfort when they do not have their customary parent or caretaker with them on a regular basis, when despite their cries, this person does not come back. The baby can feel dysregulated both emotionally and physiologically if their normal routines are not carried out by their familiar person; they yearn to be with that person and they want desperately to regain the familiar feelings of being with that person.

At this age, the loss of a parent or a primary caretaker represents an enormous disruption for the infant and may, at least temporarily, cause distress and discomfort and interrupt development. It may also affect the degree of trust, security, and comfort the baby feels in subsequent relationships.

The best way to care for an infant at this age in the absence of the primary caretaker is, as mentioned, to try to have one or two people take over her care, to try to keep to the routines of the primary caretaker and to provide a low stimulus environment to the extent possible. You will read more about how to do this in part 2 of the book.

When a parent or primary caretaker dies or is ill, there will of course be a period of chaos. If the infant can be protected from the inevitable disorganization of the household and if she can be kept apart from the most dramatic displays of sadness, while still being kept in the familiar home environment, this will be best.

Older Infants to Young Toddlers (One to Two Years)

Diane was nineteen months old when her mother died by suicide. At the time of her mother's death, Diane's care was taken over by a beloved housekeeper, who noticed that Diane was more fussy than usual, often asked for her mother and was hard to soothe. Diane had trouble going down for naps, and she stopped sleeping through the night, which she had previously been able to do.

When Diane was four years old, her father took her to a psychoanalyst for help. In working with Diane through play therapy, her analyst learned that Diane felt that she herself had been the cause of her mother's disappearance, and she had many wishful ideas that she could somehow bring her mother back.[17]

Starting in toddlerhood, most children are quite aware of changes in their environment. If a close family member becomes ill or dies, even toddlers will be aware of the absence of the person, and they will also register the different moods of other family members as they experience sadness and grief. This will be true even if the person who has been lost is not the primary caretaker.

Toddlers will also be acutely affected by the changes in their routine and environment that often accompany the death of a family member. Everything may feel strange and different for quite a while.

Even a one-year-old notices when Mommy or Daddy is different. They are not able to understand verbal language entirely, but they do understand and take in the feeling states of those around them.

If a loss has occurred in the family—for example, if a parent or a beloved grandparent or sibling has died—a one-year-old will notice their absence. They will feel sad or anxious or angry when that person does not reappear. If they had a positive attachment with that person, they will long for them to come back, and they may search for them in all the familiar places.

Toddlers of this age may even blame themselves for the loss. The one-and-a-half-year-old cannot understand where a loved one who has died has gone and why they are not coming back. As a result, they are prone to developing fantasies related to the disappearance of a loved one, just as Diane did. Because their language skills are very limited, they also can neither express their worries about where their loved one is nor understand all of what is said to them about this. However, they still need the adults around them to explain what has happened. And they need to hear this explanation repeatedly and throughout their childhood. This is because they may not be able to hold on to the reality of what has happened and may revert to fantasy. Just as the adults who care for the young toddler need to repeatedly tell the story of what has happened, they also need to be able to answer all the questions that come up around the loss as the toddler gets older and is able to ask more questions.

Toddlers (Two to Three Years)

In his autobiographical novel, *A Death in the Family*, James Agee narrates the experience of loss for a three-year-old. Catherine was three when her father died and her mother went into mourning. Catherine's care was temporarily taken over by her five-year-old brother, Rufus, and her aunt. Agee wrote, "Catherine did not like being buttoned up by Rufus or being bossed around by him, and breakfast wasn't like breakfast either. . . . Everything was (strange), (the house) was so still and it seemed dark."[18]

At three, Catherine felt the change in her routine and her environment. Having her brother help her dress was new and unpleasant. Her aunt's way of preparing breakfast was clearly not like her mother's, and the lack of conversation at breakfast was different from the usual. She experienced the changes in her household by feeling uncomfortable, and she also experienced them on a bodily level: she was not hungry, and even if she ate, things tasted different.

This is typical of the toddler and young child. We know that the young toddler feels sad when someone she loves leaves—and it is commonplace to see her experience angry feelings when someone she loves does not come to her when she wants them. When a toddler loses a loved one, this sadness and anger may come and go, but it can persist over days, weeks, and months. The toddler may feel uncomfortable and annoyed by all the differences in her life and she may yearn for the return of her lost loved one.

This is the age at which the child can begin to experience grief and mourning.

The two-to-three-year-old understands that people leave, and she does not like it when they do. But she does not understand that someone can leave her because they have died. In her mind, someone leaves because they want to, and if someone in her life dies, she may worry that they have left because she was bad or unlovable.

As any babysitter knows, when a toddler's mother goes out the door, the toddler begins to cry. And if her mother does not come back immediately after she starts crying, she continues to cry, and she does not understand why her mother does not return. She may be able to be soothed and reassured and to stop crying after a few minutes, but crying is usually her first response. She is sad when her mother leaves her—and she is angry.

At this age, the toddler is very strong-minded and stubborn. She is becoming her own person, with her own opinions. Autonomy is important to her, and she wants to do what she wants to do, when she wants to do it. If she wants to feed herself or zip up her own jacket, you will have a fight on your hands if you try to interfere! At this age, the toddler wants to gain control over what she does and where she goes. She does not like to be told no, and she herself will often say no when asked or told to do something, no matter how reasonable the request may be. When the toddler feels that she is not in control, she rebels, wanting to regain a sense of power.

On the other hand, when the toddler feels in control, she is on top of the world.

So, if a toddler wants her mother and she does not come, whether because she has left the house, gone on a prolonged trip, become ill, or, in the worst case, has died, the toddler will feel very upset. If she has the repeated experience of wanting and yearning for her mother (in the case of a prolonged absence or death), this upset can last for days, weeks, or months.

What's more, from around one and a half to three years of age, the toddler believes that she controls what happens in her world. She truly believes that if a good thing happens, it is her doing, and if a bad thing happens, it is also her doing. This leads her to think that if a parent or other loved one leaves—whether briefly or forever—it is her fault.

This sense of having caused her own abandonment is destructive. It can have long-lasting effects on her sense of self. She may feel bad and unlovable.

When a parent or other loved one leaves, the child of this age can experience sadness, yearning, frustration, and anger. They *want* to be with the people they love, and they do not want them to leave!

Toddlers of this age have been observed to follow a predictable pattern when separated from their mothers or primary caretakers for two weeks or more, especially when an adequate substitute caretaker is not available. John Bowlby observed toddlers in orphanages and hospitals who lost their mothers and described what happened.[19] The children in the hospital were ill themselves and did not have access to their mothers during their hospital stays, and those in the orphanages had lost their mothers, either temporarily or permanently.

Bowlby observed the toddlers going through a series of feelings, which he named protest, despair, and detachment.

He noted that protest can last from a few hours to seven or eight days and that it is characterized by demonstrations of anger, including crying, rattling the bars of the crib, and throwing any toys or books available. He said that the child has a strong desire for the lost parent and the expectation—based on previous experience—that they will respond to her cries. When they do not, the child may feel acutely anxious, confused, and frightened.

After protest comes what Bowlby termed despair, a time that is characterized by the toddler's continuing desire for the parent accompanied by increasing hopelessness that the parent will return. The active physical demonstrations of anger and frustration diminish when a toddler enters this phase, and her crying becomes monotonous and sporadic. The child sadly becomes withdrawn and apathetic, and she makes no demands on those around her. She is in deep mourning. This is the quiet stage known to nurses and pediatricians who work in hospitals and orphanages.

Finally, detachment is the phase which Bowlby described as gradually following despair. During this phase, the child stops crying and shows more interest in her environment. Because of this, those caring for the child may believe that the child is recovering. However, Bowlby noted that this is not the case. For the child who has been left by a parent or other beloved caretaker, this is a defensive device for coping with distress. The child is actually in the process of detaching from her own need for love and attachment, a very worrisome and undesirable process indeed.

We rarely see despair or detachment in children who are kept at home or are placed in a loving substitute home after a loss. But if you do see signs of either of these phases, it is an important indication that the toddler is suffering too much and needs immediate help.

When the period of detachment continues to the point that desire for the primary caretaker or any kind of intimate maternal care disappears, this is extremely serious and includes the possibility that the child will develop more permanent detachment from relationships with others or what we now call a reactive attachment disorder.

Bowlby's work shows how children from two years of age onward are affected by the longer-term loss of a parent or beloved caretaker, especially when a good substitute caretaker is not provided.

What is also important about Bowlby's work is that he proved beyond a doubt that even the youngest of children can experience longing, sadness, anger, anxiety, and despair when separated from their parents, something that was not believed or taken into consideration before he did his research.

He also showed that the length of the separation (in part) determines the response of the child—with longer periods of loss accompanied by the lack of an adequate substitute caretaker leading to the poorest outcomes—including the reaction he described as detachment.

Bowlby's studies also shed light on what happens when children of this age are reunited with parents after prolonged separations (two weeks or more). He said that children between one and four years of age experience a "tumultuous mixture of desire and anger" when they see their parents again. They may turn their heads and refuse to look at their parent. They may refuse hugs, and they may seem as if they cannot even hear what their parent is saying to them.

However, it will be reassuring to parents to know that Bowlby found that even after absences of several weeks the toddlers he observed were able to maintain a strong attachment to their parents. He stated, "Although the feeling they had for their parents was confused and compounded by extremes of love, demand and hostility, a strong relationship remained."

A lesser version of this reaction is something that parents who leave their toddlers at daycare are familiar with. After a long day, some toddlers will keep playing when the parent walks into the room to pick them up, ignoring the parent's presence. Often parents feel hurt and confused by this reaction, but it is important for them to understand that this is just their child's way of expressing their mixed feelings about having been left. Some little ones may have tried to tamp down their need for their parent in order to get along during the day—and it may take a few minutes to reconnect to their parents. Others may be angry at having been left and may show this by ignoring the parent or refusing to look at them.

Three to Four Years Old

While three-year-old Marco and his mother were watching TV one Sunday morning, his mother started to feel unwell. She told him to go get his father, and he ran out of the room to do so. When he and his father arrived back in the room, Marco's mother said she was feeling terrible and she didn't know what was wrong. She asked her husband to call 911. As Marco watched, the EMTs came, examined his mother, attached leads to her chest, did an EKG, and announced that she was having a heart attack. They carried his mother out on a gurney, and Marco looked on as she left in the ambulance.

Marco did not cry then or when he was left with the next-door neighbor. He did not cry when his grandmother came to pick him up a few hours later or when his father came home that night without his mother.

Was Marco grieving? Did he miss his mother or wonder what had happened to her?

Of course.

But at three years old, Marco was not yet able to give his feelings words.

What did happen later that night as he went to sleep is that he asked for Mommy. He wanted to know where she was.

At three, Marco did not know about hospitals. He did not know what a heart attack was. All he knew was that Mommy was not there and that she had gone off in a big white van with a siren.

He missed her. But even saying that was a bit beyond his ability.

For the entire time that his mother was in the hospital—and in fact for months and years afterward—Marco played with his ambulances and his fire trucks. He had his father think up scenarios where someone was in trouble and needed to be saved. And then Marco would come to the rescue with his little ambulance or truck.

This was Marco's way of working out what had happened to his mother. He struggled for quite a long time to understand that she had been in trouble and that the men in the ambulance had "saved" her. It had been excruciating for him to stand by helplessly as his mother was taken away and he fervently wished he could have helped her.

This was an experience like none Marco had ever had; it had happened suddenly, it had been scary, and it had been overwhelming to him. It took him a long time to understand the events of that Sunday morning and to accept that someone he loved could suddenly be taken away and there was nothing he could do about it.

For Marco, grief came in the form of confusion and intense missing feelings. He tried to work out what he felt and saw. Mostly, he did this through his play. He played out what he remembered of the event, and he elaborated and had his father elaborate on these memories. He worked and worked to understand what had happened.

The three-year-old understands the world in a very limited way. He still interprets everything from a me-centered point of view. So, for example, if someone leaves or dies, he is prone to interpreting this as resulting from something he did—or didn't do, much like the younger toddler. Marco might have worried that his mother left because he had taken a penny from the store "give a penny take a penny" bowl the day before and she had been annoyed with him about this.

Three-year-olds also have a very limited understanding of illness and death. It is very hard for them to understand where someone has gone if they are in the hospital or if they have died. They may ask the same questions over and over again, even after an explanation has been given to them. They need the adults around them to explain carefully and factually what has happened—and to do so as often as they ask about the whereabouts of their loved one or when they're coming back. In Marco's case, both his grandmother and his father told him that Mommy had become very sick and that the doctors were trying to help her at the hospital.

Three-year-olds also need to see grief modeled in appropriate ways. Marco's father was afraid to cry in front of Marco—but in fact, when Marco did see him crying a few days after his mother was hospitalized, Marco himself was able to begin to cry. While he was crying, his father told Marco that he missed Marco's mother very much and that he was worried about her. This helped Marco to be able to cry and to find the words about his own missing and worried feelings.

The three-year-old is also prone to generalizing from one experience to others. As a result, a three-year-old who has lost a relative to death, illness, or abandonment is likely to worry that other adults will also go away. They need frequent reassurance that this is not going to happen any time in the near future (if this is true, of course).

Four to Five Years Old

Jacky was four when his father died by suicide. His mother went down to the basement and discovered his father hanging from an overhead pipe. She did not know if Jacky had come down behind her or if he had stayed upstairs, but several days after his father's death Jacky's mother noticed that Jacky had become afraid of going down to the basement and he was also especially fearful at bedtime.

When Jacky's grandmother brought him to see me, the first thing he did when he got into my playroom was to sit down in front of the dollhouse. He looked at all the little figures, chose the "daddy" doll, and threw him behind the house. When I asked, "What happened to daddy?" he retrieved the figure, put him on top of the house, and said, "Daddy's on the roof."

This is how Jacky's grandmother found out that when his grandfather had said to Jacky that his father was "up there" (meaning heaven), Jacky thought that his father had just gone to live on the roof of the house.

Jacky was grieving, but in his case, his initial grief was expressed through fearfulness and misunderstanding. Once I helped Jacky to understand that his daddy had died and could not come back, other emotions emerged: he was angry at God for taking his father, he missed his dad, and he needed a great deal more snuggling time with his mother. He was not able to say that he was sad, but this seemed evident the many times he put his head in his mother's lap or went to her for extra cuddles during our sessions.

The four-to-five-year-old child is in some ways much more like an older child. He is generally sociable, interested in all sorts of activities, and well connected to both father and mother. When the four-year-old suffers a separation or loss, he is like older children in his awareness of the loss; he will generally ask more questions and be able to understand more about the reasons for the separation. But, like the three-year-old, he will still have misconceptions about what happened and why and will need frequent reminders from adults about the facts. He will still be confused at times about where his loved one has gone and why they are not coming back.

The question of whether there is an afterlife may be important to the four-to-five-year-old. He may imagine that his loved one lives on in heaven and is able to see and hear him. This concept is double-edged—on the one hand, it may be comforting for the five-year-old to believe in the ongoing presence of his loved one, and on the other hand, it may be frightening to imagine the loved one can see him at all times, even when he is doing things he knows he shouldn't.

Rufus was the five-year-old beautifully described by James Agee in his novel, *A Death in the Family.*[20] Agee was adept at describing the innermost thoughts of this child. He described what Rufus thought after he had told some older boys about his father's death: "He felt so uneasy, deep inside his stomach, that he could not think about it anymore. He wished he hadn't done it, he wished he could go back and not do anything of the kind."[21] Rufus wished his father could know what he had done and just tell him that what he was done was bad. At the same time he wished that his father could tell him that it was OK and he understood that he had not meant to be bad. Rufus worried that his father's soul could see him from heaven and that made him feel helpless. He couldn't talk to his father's soul, he couldn't defend himself, and worst of all, he couldn't hide from a soul. He worried that his father's soul was ashamed of him.

It is common for the child of this age to feel that they are bad or that they were bad when their loved one was still alive and to imagine their lost loved one being critical of them.

Four-to-five-year-olds, like children of all ages, have a profound need for love and affection. If the person who died was a parent or close relative, their sad, missing, and longing feelings will be profound.

Séamas O'Reilly, whose mother died when he was five, poignantly described a dream he had after her death in which he saw his mother: "I just want to reach her so I can be held and so I can tell her that I want her to be back . . . I want to tell her that I'm sad and I don't understand, and that none of this makes any sense . . . I just want her to hold me in the way of living people . . . I'm just trying to get to her, trying to make it to the point where she can pick me up, where I can sit on her lap and feel her close and know again how it is to be held by someone whose heart isn't breaking."[22]

It is not unusual for four-to-five-year-olds to have wishful dreams and fantasies that they reunite with their lost loved one. These dreams and fantasies can be both comforting and, when the child wakes up, profoundly painful. In fact, this can happen to people of any age, and many adults report having the same experience.

The four-to-five-year-old is still a small child whose feelings of missing a loved one are visceral; they feel their feelings in their bodies, through stomachaches or headaches or a loss of appetite or difficulty sleeping. Their memories of the lost loved one will often involve touch and holding—and these are some of the things they may miss the most.

At night, in the dark, children worry about separation of all kinds. Going to sleep can feel like a separation—and after experiencing a loss, the separation at night may feel extra scary. At bedtime, children may ask a parent if the parent is going to die, if a sibling is going to die, if their teacher or other familiar person is going to die. And while none of us know for sure how long we will live, it is best to reassure the child that most people live to an old age.

It can also be helpful for parents to talk about all the ways they take care of themselves to make sure that they live a long, long life.

Six to Eleven Years Old

When Maddie was nine, she was a fun-loving, gregarious girl. She did well in school and had lots of friends. That year her mother began feeling tired, and she had some aches and pains, but nothing specific. Maddie was not fazed by her mother's minor complaints.

And then during the summer, when things quieted down with her three children, Maddie's mother took the time to go to her family doctor and her gynecologist to have her symptoms investigated. She was sent for a scan and was shocked to receive a diagnosis of stage 3 ovarian cancer.

Maddie's mother began chemotherapy right away and was not sure what to say to her children about all of this. Her husband wanted to shield the children from the diagnosis, so at first all they told the children was that mom was sick and needed to go to the hospital each day to receive her medication.

At nine, Maddie, the oldest, was quite aware of her parents' moods, and she quickly realized that her parents were anxious and distressed and that something serious must be wrong with her mother. At bedtime one night, shortly after her mother began treatment, she asked her mother if she had cancer. Wanting to be honest, her mother said yes. Maddie cried and cried, and she and her mother ended up sleeping together in Maddie's bed that night.

From that point on, Maddie devoted herself to helping her mother. Her attitude toward her two younger siblings changed and she became like a junior mother to them. She also asked her mother what she could do around the house, made her mother tea, and started trying to be more independent with her homework.

After six months of treatment, Maddie's mother was hospitalized for the first time. Maddie was upset and missed her mother terribly. At night she cried in her room, and when her father came in to say good-night and found her crying, he just did not know what to do. He sat with her and told her that he was sad too—but he really could not tolerate going too deeply into his own feelings, so great was his distress over his wife's illness.

When Maddie was ten, it became clear that her mother's cancer was progressing. Maddie asked her mother if she was going to die, and her mother broke down crying. At this point Maddie's mother was physically very weak and did not have the psychological resources to answer this question.

But Maddie knew the answer from her mother's response.

Maddie's mother was now sleeping in the living room in a hospital bed, and Maddie insisted on sleeping on the couch nearby. She made cards for her mother almost every day, and she hated it when the social worker came by to talk with her and her brothers. Maddie wanted nothing to do with this woman and ran up to her room as the social worker talked to the younger children.

By this time, Maddie was receiving all Cs at school. She had stopped seeing her friends on the weekends, and she was much quieter even when she was around her old friends at school.

This is what Maggie's grief looked like.

Maggie used her energy to help her mother and to try to make her mother happy.

Maggie was very sad and she understood what the future held.

Maddie was with her mother when she died. She sat next to her mother's bed with her father and her brothers, and she held her mother's hand.

After the emergency services were called, Maddie continued to sit in the chair by her mother's bed. And when the EMS workers took her mother's body out of the house, Maddie barely moved and she spoke to no one.

This is also what Maddie's grief looked like. As much as she had anticipated her mother's death, when it finally came, she was shocked into immobility. She sat motionless and silent, much as I had when my own father died.

In the weeks following her mother's death, Maddie attended the funeral and returned to school. She continued to help take care of her younger siblings, and she also helped her father around the house. One night her father saw her curled up in her brother's bed, rocking her younger brother to sleep. Maddie was comforting her younger brother as she remembered her mother comforting her. She comforted her younger brother as she *wanted* to still be comforted herself. She turned her wish to be comforted into an effort to comfort and help others.

This is one way the six-to-eleven-year-old can respond to grief. But there are many other ways as well. Some children of this age can show their grief directly by looking sad, crying, and talking about their sadness. Some do not show their grief in obvious ways, but it can be seen indirectly in their play activities, drawings, moods, or behavior.

Maddie was also one of these. She had trouble expressing her grief directly. Instead, she took care of her mother and her siblings. And after her mother's death, she took special pleasure in comforting her younger brothers.

As you can see from the example of Maddie, the child of six to eleven is able to experience grief in all of its manifestations. With appropriate support, the child of this age will be able both to mourn and to understand the full meaning of her loss. Like the younger child, she will miss her loved one intensely, and she will dip in and out of these missing feelings. But she will also have a greater capacity than the younger child to understand the significance and permanence of the loss, to review her memories of her loved one, and to experience the pain of realizing that they will never come back.

Older children in this age range, around ten and eleven, may or may not show their sadness openly. They may keep some of their feelings so private that adults close to them may wonder if they are indeed sad at all. They may attempt to keep up a good face and to proceed with life as if nothing has happened. At this age, children do not want to be different from their friends, and they often do not want to talk about their difficult feelings. Crying may be hard for them as it can be associated with being a baby, something the ten-to-eleven-year-old does not want to be.

But one way that grief or the feelings around loss may be expressed by children of this age is through the body, just like younger children and babies. Stomachaches, headaches, difficulty sleeping, sleeping too much, clumsiness, repeated accidents or illnesses, or pleas to stay home from school may indicate that the child is having difficult feelings. When she is not able to talk about her feelings, it can be helpful for a parent, teacher, pediatrician, or school nurse to suggest that some of these bodily feelings might have to do with being sad. Some children will be relieved to learn this—while others may vehemently object!

Normally, the child of this age is actively engaged with school and friends. She has become very interested in life beyond the family.

Outside interests such as video games, social media, sports, clubs, dance, musical instrument practice, or other activities will often consume much of her time. However, this does not mean that she does not need the love and presence of her parents, teachers, and friends to help her to feel safe, secure, and motivated to achieve.

Loss at this age can be devastating to the child, and any diminution of demonstrated feeling cannot be taken as indicating that she is any less sad or any less affected than the younger child.

Children of this age may also show their sadness or preoccupation through difficulties at school. Concentration may be interrupted, and the child's academic work may suffer. The child may be preoccupied by sad feelings or by memories of their lost loved one or by thoughts about what happened to their lost one. Patience and understanding on the part of teachers and parents is crucial when this happens. The child may also need help learning how to allow herself time to have feelings as well as time to concentrate on schoolwork. Helping the child to take breaks when needed and then to get back to work may be useful. Having a safe space at school for the child to go to when she is feeling particularly sad may also be helpful.

Relationships with friends may suffer. A child who has experienced loss may withdraw from friends for a while. Again, help from parents and teachers is important. The child may feel "weird" or "different" and may need help reintegrating into their classroom or their friend group.

Preteens (Eleven to Twelve Years Old)

Raj was eleven and a half when his parents separated, and his father went to live and work in India. Raj refused to talk to his mother about how he felt about his parents' separation, but she noticed him being harder on himself. When he couldn't do something on the first or second try, he berated himself. When he wasn't chosen for the travel team, he talked about how much he sucked at soccer.

Previously, Raj had been an easygoing boy. His mother was now worried about him and brought him to see me.

Through therapy for Raj, and meetings with the mother, I helped them both to understand that Raj blamed himself for his father's departure. While he did not think that he caused his parent's separation, he did think that if had been good enough, if his father had loved him enough, his father would have stayed in the United States rather than going to India.

It is difficult for children to understand why a parent would leave them voluntarily. When a parent or a sibling leaves the home or, even worse, if they die by suicide, children of all ages can feel that they were not worthy of love, that they were not good enough to keep the parent or sibling around, or that they were so bad that the parent or sibling left.

The preteen is at an especially precarious stage of life—leaving childhood behind and just waiting to embark on being a teen. Sometimes the child of this age behaves like the younger version of themselves and sometimes they seem like they are already teenagers. This is because they are in conflict—although they may not admit it. Sometimes they want to be a child and be taken care of and sometimes they want to be more like a teenager and do as they please. Often they toggle between these two positions on a moment to moment basis.

At this age, school, friends, social media, and activities are particularly important. What friends are doing may at times be more important than what parents say. What is happening online, at school, and with friends becomes the focus of attention over family life.

When a child of this age loses a loved one, feelings of sadness and grief may be held inside because the preteen is afraid of the regression that may occur if they let themselves feel too sad. They may fear that crying will make them look babyish. They may also worry about being different from their friends. If a parent or a sibling dies, they may worry that their friends will think that this is strange and that *they* are strange. At the same time, they may feel a bit alienated from their friends because they *are* different now.

No matter what they say or how they seem after a loss, the eleven-to-twelve-year-old still needs all the love and concern that the younger child needs. While it may not feel so good to them, talking about their feelings and even crying can be encouraged.

The Teen Years (Thirteen to Twenty)

Coco was fourteen when her grandfather died suddenly of Covid-19. A few days later her mother and her sister tested positive for Covid as well. Coco was sent to her aunt's house while her mother and sister stayed at home and took care of each other. Coco missed her grandfather terribly, and on top of that, she missed her mother and her sister. She was desperate to go home to take care of them and often begged her aunt to allow her to go. While at her aunt's, Coco stayed on the couch much of the time, skipping many of her online classes, and mostly just checking social media. She did very little of her homework and spent a great deal of time complaining to her aunt about her friends.

Coco was old enough to grieve her grandfather's death much as an adult would. However, the suddenness of his illness and death and the illness of her mother and sister immediately following his death interfered with her ability to mourn properly and to proceed with her daily life in a productive fashion.

When there are external factors such as financial difficulties or a move that get in the way of a normal grief process, children of all ages are at risk for trouble in their mourning, including developing delayed or disordered mourning. (We will talk more about this in part 2).

Coco had so many painful events in a row that she became overwhelmed. She lost her grandfather, she worried about her mother and sister being ill, and she moved to a new home all in the space of two weeks.

Coco had trouble attending online class and doing her online schoolwork. She was preoccupied and worried. She also felt weird. She had lost her grandfather and she was living in a new place. She worried that the other kids in online class would see the new background of her aunt's house and wonder where she was and why she had been missing from class for so many days. She felt different than she had before her grandfather died, and she was worried that other kids would notice.

Coco's experience illustrates the way many older children and teens feel. They don't want to feel—or be—different from their friends. When they suffer a loss, they sometimes feel like others look at them differently. And when their friends don't reach out to them following the loss, or if their friends avoid the subject of the loss or seem awkward around them because they don't know what to say, the teen often interprets this as their friends not caring.

For another example, Christine was seventeen when her sister was killed by a drunk driver. Christine blamed herself and said over and over that she should have been with her sister that night—and if she had been, her sister would still be alive.

It is not unusual for children of any age to blame themselves for the death of a loved one. Depending on their age and stage of development, this self-blame will take different forms. As we talked about before, the very young child may imagine that the loved one left because they were bad. Older children may feel that they were not smart enough or lovable enough for the sibling or the parent to stay alive for them. Still older children and teens may worry that they did not do all they should have done for the loved one or that they did things they should not have done and thus contributed to the loss.

Christine, for example, felt that if only she had decided to go with her sister that night instead of being with her own friends, that she might, somehow, have been able to help her sister to avoid the accident. If she had invited her sister to go with her and her friends, it wouldn't have happened. Or if only she had agreed to do something with her sister that night, perhaps the timing would have been different, and they would not have been in the spot where the sister was hit when the drunk driver came down the road. This belief was tenacious. It took Christine time—and some therapy—to begin to consider the possibility that the accident was not in any way her fault.

Teenagers can mourn much as adults can, but it is important to remember that they are still in the process of development. They still need a great deal of help and support after a loss. If a parent or close relative dies or leaves, the teenager's development will be affected. While they may be more independent and more capable than younger children, teenagers still need encouragement to experience and express their feelings directly. They also still need the love, attention, guidance, limit setting, and role modeling of both parents and grandparents during their mourning, and they will be deeply affected in innumerable ways by their loss.

And in the case of the loss of a close friend, teens are particularly vulnerable.

Friends are more meaningful than ever before in the course of development, and the loss of a good friend, whether due to death or other circumstance, will be deeply painful. It may take a long time for a teen to mourn the loss of a close friend, and during this time, their feelings regarding their loss may be quite dramatic.

Another important aspect of adolescence is the fact that teens are in the process of forming their identities. Close relatives, especially parents and grandparents as well as close friends, provide models for teens either to identify with or to disidentify with. In other words, teenagers may choose (consciously or unconsciously) to be like a parent, grandparent, or friend or they may choose to be different from them. For example, a teen who dislikes a certain characteristic of her mother's may vow never to be that way herself. This decision will be part of her identity in terms of how she presents herself to the world and how she defines herself.

Teens are also in the process of working out how relationships work. They will observe their parents' relationship and their parents' relationships with other people, and that will provide a powerful basis for what they understand intimate relationships and friendships to be. If a parent is lost, the opportunity for continued observation of the parental relationship and the relationships the parent has with others is lost.

Also lost are all the interactions the teen might have had with the parent or other loved one over the course of later teen years and early adulthood. And this is important—because these interactions serve as a way for the teen to work on and work through their mixed feelings, their idealizations, and their tendency to devalue those close to them.

Teens have their own relationships with each parent and each close relative, and these relationships are important. They are practice grounds for future relationships. They are templates upon which the teen may model future relationships.

For example, the teenage girl needs her father (and grandfather and uncles) and her relationships with them in order to understand and practice how to relate to men. How her male relatives treat her will form an important basis for how she understands male-female patterns of relatedness and what she expects from the men in her life going forward.

If her father (or close grandfather or uncle) should die during her teen years, she not only loses an important relationship, but as mentioned, she also loses an infinite number of opportunities for interaction and further development in negotiating relationships with men.

To be more specific, the young child idealizes most adults, especially their parents. When children are under the age of seven or eight, they often see their parents and grandparents as knowing everything and being able to do anything. As children get older, they begin to see that their parents and older relatives may not actually know it all, and they see that they may have areas of weakness and incompetence. By adolescence, teens often become quite critical of their older relatives, especially their parents, and there may be a prolonged period where disagreements are common.

It may take until the early to late twenties for children to recognize that their parents aren't actually wrong all the time—and to appreciate what their parents have provided for them. If a parent should be lost before young adulthood, the child or teen is deprived of the opportunity to fully work out her image of her parent and her relationship with them. Idealization or devaluation of the parent who died may persist, and it may be hard to work through these without the help of either a great deal of introspection or actual therapy.

In sum, the loss of a parent, close friend, or loved one in adolescence is an event of extreme importance. The teen may be able to mourn and grieve much like an adult but, at the same time, her feelings about life, about herself, about relationships and, in fact, her overall development may be affected in numerous important ways.

The Loss of a Loved One

In this chapter, I talk about the loss of a parent, grandparent, sibling, friend, or pet and the various ways these losses may be experienced by children and teens.

In chapter 4, I talk about how the manner of loss, whether through divorce, illness, violence, war, or suicide, can affect children. And in chapter 5, I talk about what has been called "ambiguous loss," which is the kind of loss that is often not recognized as such.

With the information provided here, you will understand how each kind of loss may affect the child in your life. After each kind of loss I also include a short section called "Continuing Connections." Following a significant loss, children (and others) find ways to hold on to aspects of the person they have lost. This is a crucial part of grief and mourning because, for many, to entirely give up someone who has been so loved is just too difficult a task. Reading these sections will help you to understand what otherwise might seem like unusual behavior or preferences in children who have experienced loss.

The Loss of a Parent

The loss of a parent, whether due to death or estrangement, is a blow like no other. When a parent dies or leaves, the child is in a unique situation because of the special nature of her tie to her parent and her real and ongoing need for the love and care that the parent provided—or could have provided.

A child who loses a parent will never be the same. They will be affected in innumerable ways by their loss, and they will always feel different from those who did not lose a parent early in life.

The effects of such a loss are lifelong—they will shape how the child sees herself, how she views life, how she feels about relationships, and how she relates to others.

This was certainly true for me.

My father was the kind of person who could take over a room within minutes of arriving. He was larger than life—literally. At six foot two, and two hundred and fifty pounds or so, people noticed him. This was partially because of his size, but it was also because he was good at connecting with people and he knew how to tell a joke.

When my father and mother came to visit me at summer camp on Parent's Day each year, my father loved to schmooze with the counselors, having once been a camp counselor himself. But the year I remember the most was the year he didn't come.

My father had died in March, and when my mother came to visit me at camp in July, she came alone. It was a rainy day so my mother and I just sat in the car. We barely spoke. It was such a different visit. While my father had chatted up everyone around him, my mother sat quietly, just with me, asking about camp. Before leaving, she handed me a tin of brownies, her way of expressing love. And while we did not mention his absence, I realize now that we were both missing my father and his enormous, larger than life presence.

I had many other opportunities to miss my father, of course. When we studied Soviet-American relations my senior year in high school, I found myself wishing I had asked my father more about his trip to Russia. When other people talked about their grandparents, I wished I had asked him more about his parents, whom I had never met. When I wondered about his childhood, I realized I knew very little and wished he had told me more. Over all the years of my adolescence, when I felt lonely or sad or in need of advice, I missed him.

However, whenever my father gave me advice, he would say, "I think you should do X . . . but do what you want," putting me in the difficult position of knowing what he thought and being given permission to do what I wanted—all at the same time. He made it look as if he were giving me freedom, but the problem was that he also let me know that he would disapprove if I chose an option different from what he suggested. This was one of his favorite tricks.

Following his death, there were many occasions when I would have liked to ask my father his opinion—but at the same time, I realize that I would have probably chosen to ignore it. It is also true that it was hard not to have any advice given at all (my mother was not one to tell anyone what to do). I felt too responsible for myself after my father's death, and sometimes I just needed someone else to decide something for me—or to provide an opinion I could push back against.

My mother had always deferred to my father, and she had never really been helpful to me in making decisions. So after my father died, I didn't really have a parent to lean on for guidance.

I think missing my father was sometimes about feeling rudderless—not knowing which way to go. At least hearing his opinion would have given me some sense of direction—even if I would have chosen to reject it, argue with him about it, or do the opposite of what he advised.

After my father died I had so much control and authority over my own life—it was really too much. On the one hand, I loved the freedom and autonomy, but on the other hand, it was terrifying. These mixed feelings continued through early adulthood. My missing feelings were sometimes a deep ache, sometimes a feeling of anxiety, and other times they were disguised as feelings of false security.

I often wondered what my father would think of what I was doing and whether he would be proud or disapproving.

Even now, as a mature adult, I still wonder. And I still miss him. When my son graduated from college last year, I thought about my father. I imagined how proud he would have been of this grandson, and I thought about how much my son missed never knowing his grandfather. On occasions like this, it is impossible not to miss my father.

It is a universal truth that no loss deprives a child of so much opportunity to love and be loved as the loss of a parent. And it is also true that no loss requires such a difficult task of adaptation.

When a child loses a parent, her life is irrevocably changed. She is suddenly and violently transported to a place made up of unknowns: Where will I find love now that my parent is gone? Who will take care of me? Who am I now without my parent? How can I go on without them? What if my other parent dies?

There are so many questions—and for long periods of time, there are no answers.

While an adult distributes love among any number of meaningful relationships—their spouse or partner, their parents, their children, their siblings, their friends—the child, especially the very young child, invests almost all of her love in her parents.

The loss of a parent is also particularly hard because the relationship between child and parent is the most critical of all formative relationships in a child's life. It is the wellspring from which love comes, and it is the model for all future relationships.[1]

While the relationship between parent and child may not have been perfect, it is nonetheless the relationship she will refer to in her mind when evaluating other relationships for the rest of her life. The death of a parent interrupts childhood and cannot help but transform the child. It will affect her development, her sense of self, her future relationships, and her psychological health. Who she might have been is forever altered by this loss and its impact.

She mourns what she lost, and she mourns what her parent lost in not getting to know her as she grew up.

Teigan, a young adult I met through Winston's Wish and Apart of Me, talked with me about this. She described what it felt like to experience the passing of time after her mother's death and how she came to recognize the magnitude of her loss. She said, "The idea of time terrifies me; every anniversary as I grow older I'm moving away from my mum. It was just nine years ago; it freaks me out . . . it's still going to impact me no matter how many years it's been . . . also as it gets longer I'm afraid people will forget her. It's my responsibility to talk about her and remember her. . . . and I'm grieving for [myself too, for] the person she didn't get to meet—that's a big thing."

Most people who lose a parent in childhood remember the exact moment they found out that their parent was going to die or the moment they found out that their parent had died. As Maxine Harris says in her book, *The Loss That Is Forever*, personal time becomes marked in terms of "before" and "after."[2]

Teigan remembers the night she found out that she was going to lose her mother. Her mother was cooking and kept burning herself. Her father realized something was very wrong and called an ambulance. That night they learned that her mother had a malignant brain tumor.

Teigan was eleven when her mother died and she was fully aware of what was happening throughout her mother's diagnosis, treatment, and eventual decline. She described for me how different her life was after her mother died, how different her father was and how difficult it was when he decided to begin dating again. Just about everything felt different about her life.

The novelist James Agee describes the feelings that young children have immediately following loss so well in his book *A Death in the Family*. He says this about five-year-old Rufus and his three-year-old sister on the day of their father's funeral:

> The house echoed, and there was still an extraordinary fragrance of carnations. Their mother was in the East Room. "My darlings," she said; she looked as if she had traveled a great distance, and now they knew that everything had changed. They put their heads against her, still knowing that nothing would ever be the same again, and she caught them so close they could smell her, and they loved her, but it made no difference. She could not say anything, and neither could they . . . and now instead of love for her they felt sadness.[3]

As Agee illustrates, the loss of a parent is also particularly hard because the loss powerfully affects the remaining parent. Not only does the child lose one parent, but often the other parent retreats into grief and the child loses that parent too, at least for a period of time. This can be called ambiguous loss, which we'll explore more in chapter 5.

It is helpful to consider the age and stage of development of the child when the loss of a parent occurs in order to understand how the child will experience the loss and how the loss will affect the child.

Even the youngest infant who loses her parent, particularly if the parent was the primary caretaker, will be enormously affected. As described in chapter 2, while the infant is completely unable to understand the concepts of separation and death, she will feel the difference in caretaking after the loss of a parent. When others take over her care, familiar rhythms and routines of caretaking will be absent and new ones will take their place.

The infant may react to these differences with discomfort and displeasure. She may react with bodily distress and physiological dysregulation, including difficulties with sleeping and eating, and with difficulties being soothed and comforted. These reactions may last for days, weeks, or months.

But what determines how fast the baby will adjust?

Factors both internal and external to the infant will affect her adaptation. If the infant is more flexible and more resilient, and if the caregivers who come to take care of her are sensitive and competent, she may adjust after just a few days or weeks.

On the other hand, if the infant is sensitive to change, if she particularly preferred the caretaker she lost to others, and/or if she does not have access to one or two regular, sensitive caretakers following her loss, she may be more upset for a longer period of time and the effects of loss may be particularly long lasting for her.

And how about the toddler?

As detailed earlier in the book, toddlers are already extremely attached to their primary caretaker. At this age, one person simply cannot substitute for another. If, between ages one and two, a toddler loses her mother or primary caretaker, this will be a major loss, and the effects will be lifelong. At the time of the loss she will not understand the implications; she will not understand that her caretaker will not and cannot come back—but she will suffer their absence each and every day.

Older children, from ages two to eight, will understand better that the parent is really gone. They will be terribly bereft. It is inevitable that fantasies will develop about why their parent left or died. Often children of this age truly believe that the parent died because they were bad, or at least not sufficiently lovable. Often they believe that there was something they could have done to prevent their parent from dying.

Frequently children of this age will also have an enormous wish to retrieve their lost parent. Or they may want to cling to reminders of the lost parent. They may wish to die in order to go to heaven to be with their parent; they may hold on to possessions of the lost parent; they may stay loyal to the rules set down by the lost parent. They may resist any changes that other family members want to make in the home, fearing a loss of the way things were when the parent was still alive.

Keeping things as they were or keeping possessions of the lost parent can serve as a link and an important connection to the parent who died. But of course, it is not always possible to keep the home as it was for an indefinite period of time, and changes that have to be made should be introduced in a gentle way and talked about in advance and with sensitivity.

Often, children will be curious about the afterlife and may wish to believe that the lost parent is present in heaven—or even as a ghostly presence on earth. For the child who repeatedly expresses the wish to be with her parent in heaven, extra help is needed. Without such help, the possibility of suicide is real, particularly among adolescents.

The family must not be afraid to talk with the child or teen when she expresses these feelings. They must not be frightened of asking her exactly what she means, and they must be willing to ask if she has a plan to actually go to heaven. They must try to understand whether the child is expressing a feeling—a yearning to be with the parent based on missing them so intensely—or whether the child actually intends to try to get to heaven in order to be reunited with her parent.

If the child seems to be feeling particularly alone, if she seems depressed and of course, if she has a plan for how she will get to heaven, the family must seek immediate professional help—and in the interim, try to provide extra love, extra support, extra reassurance that she is valued, as well as around-the-clock monitoring of the child.

The missing feelings after a parent dies can be intense.

Again, in *A Death in the Family*, James Agee vividly describes the poignant feelings of five-year-old Rufus, who suddenly lost his father:

> He looked at his father's morsechair . . . With a sense of deep stealth and secrecy he finally went over to the chair and stood beside it. After a few moments, and after listening most intently, to be sure that no one was near, he smelled the chair, its deeply hollowed seat, the arms, the back. There was only a cold smell of tobacco and, high along the back, the smell of hair. He thought of the ash tray . . . it was empty. He ran his finger inside it; there was only a dim smudge of ash. There was nothing like enough to keep in his pocket or wrap in a paper. He looked at his finger for a moment and licked it; his tongue tasted of darkness.[4]

Rufus, like so many children who lose a parent, looked for remnants of his father—evidence of his father having been there, and reminders of what his father was like. He examined his father's favorite chair for any signs of him—whether his smell or the smell of the cigarettes he smoked. He wanted to find some leftover tobacco or some ashes to keep with him in his pocket—and he was disappointed when he found none. He tasted the tiny remnant of ashes, taking into himself what little there was left of his father.

Children who lose a parent yearn for something to hold on to or incorporate into themselves in order to keep their parent, quite literally, with them. They may adopt habits, interests, or personality traits of the lost parent or they may cherish a certain piece of furniture or clothing that was a favorite of their parent.

Children and teens may express these feelings directly or they may suffer from bodily complaints, which take the place of more direct expressions of their missing, anxious, or angry feelings. They may develop headaches, stomachaches, insomnia, or a tendency to sleep too much. They may become accident prone or worried about developing illnesses.

In his memoir, Séamas O'Reilly, whose mother died when he was five, tells a story about himself when he was ten: "Sometime in February 1996 I stopped sleeping. Each evening, a chill would settle in my stomach after I came in from school, suspending a fog of anxiety I couldn't shake."

Séamas had never had a problem with sleep before this. He wrote: "Weeks turned into months. Fatigue made me sloppy and confused in school. I grew more sullen and withdrawn, staring vacantly in class, picking at my food at mealtimes. I lost weight, and brown-beige bags grew under my eyes like coffee stains. I don't remember saying anything about any of this to my family."[5]

Eventually Séamas developed severe abdominal pain and had to be taken to his doctor. He described the doctor as "the kind of doctor who would shake a child's hand in greeting, as if you were not a ten-year-old insomniac but a city gent being shown around a country club. [He] had an outsider's insight into what was plaguing me and a doctor's knack for saying one thing while doing another."

The doctor brought out his stethoscope, poked Séamas's stomach, and said, as if they had just been talking about feelings, "Tell me, Séamas, what are you so sad about?"

"I don't want Daddy to die," Séamas replied, saying that out loud for the first time ever.

Clearly Séamas was keeping his worst fears to himself. Instead of talking about his terrible fear that his father would also die, he developed bodily signs that all was not OK with him. He had lost his mother and now he was terrified that he would also lose his father. But he could not say this to anyone—not even himself—so instead he developed stomach pains and he could not sleep at night.

And for children who lose a parent later, say in their preteen years, the loss will be just as significant as one occurring earlier in life.

As we discussed in chapter 2, the preteen is at a precarious stage of life—trying to leave childhood behind and just waiting to embark on being a teen. When a child of this age loses a parent, feelings of sadness and grief may be held inside because the child is afraid of the regression that may occur if they let themselves feel too sad. They may fear that crying will make them look babyish. They may also worry about feeling things that their friends are not feeling and about actually being different from their friends now that they have lost a parent.

No matter what they say or how they seem, after the loss of a parent, the eleven-to-twelve-year-old preteen still needs all the love and concern that the younger child needs. While it may not feel so good to them, talking about their feelings and even crying can be very important for their grief process to move forward.

As for teenagers, the loss of a parent is, as I mentioned earlier, an extremely difficult experience. Thea was thirteen when the pandemic first began in 2020. Her father was one of the early victims of Covid, before vaccination and effective treatment were available. Her father became ill, and as the days went by he became progressively shorter of breath. When it seemed that he could not catch his breath at all, Thea's mother called an ambulance. He was admitted to the hospital and put on a ventilator almost immediately; however, the support provided in the ICU was insufficient and he died three weeks later. Neither Thea nor her mother was able to see him once he went to the hospital.

Thea felt strangely removed from her father's death. He had not been that sick when she last saw him. He had been lying on the couch, asking her for drinks and snacks. And then suddenly, he was taken away and she did not see him again.

Thea was old enough to grieve her father's death much as an adult would. However, there were factors that interfered in her ability to feel all the sad and missing feelings she might have been expected to have.

The suddenness of his illness and death and the fact that she could not see him as he became more ill made it hard for the severity of his illness to feel real to her. She and her mother did not get much information about his condition, and there were very few treatment options for Covid at that point. Thea was attending school online and felt isolated. All of these factors interfered with her ability to fully accept her father's death and to experience and express the feelings that go along with grief and mourning.

Initially, Thea cried with her mother when the hospital called to say that her father had died. But after that, she found herself feeling rather numb and preferred to stay in her room, on her bed, rather than spending time with her mother. Thea had trouble doing her online schoolwork. She was preoccupied and could not concentrate. She had become more distant from her friends and did not often reach out to them over social media.

Thea's experience illustrates the way many older children and teens feel. They are profoundly affected by the loss of a parent, but they may not know how to understand or process their own feelings. For a teenager, losing a parent can be an alienating experience. Children and teens can feel different, weird, and alone. Often they don't know others who have lost a close loved one—or even if they do know someone, they are often not sure how to talk about their own feelings with them.

Teens are especially attuned to the special meaning and importance of each relationship.

Reporter Eliza Griswold wrote in the *New Yorker* about Izzy, who also lost a parent early in the pandemic. Prior to her father's death, Izzy had enjoyed wonderful late-night talks with him about everything from the nature of the universe to the book of Genesis. She said, "You don't know how alone you are until the only person who understands you isn't here."[6]

Izzy found it particularly difficult to relate to her friends after her father died. She noticed herself being short with them. "I lost my filter," Izzy said. And also, "Once you have a parent die, no one knows how to talk to you. It's awkward." Sometimes other kids raised doubts about the reality of the coronavirus. "Those conversations never end well," she said.

As I mentioned earlier, children and teens may blame themselves for a parent's death. This is endlessly troubling to them as they may feel that they played some part in the loss. They may feel they didn't do enough for their parent, or they did things they should not have done that might have caused the death. Unfortunately, guilt is common among teens who have lost a parent and may lead to a diminished sense of self-worth.

But there are other reasons for guilt as well.

When I left for college, I felt terribly guilty. Not for my father's death but for leaving my mother alone. She had never suggested that I should stay home, but I worried that she would be lonely. I was the last child in the family to go to college, and now my mother lived at home all alone.

I devised various schemes to make sure that my mother had company, volunteering my house over and over again for other students doing internships in my home city. Finally, my mother had to ask me to stop doing this, and it was only then that I realized that she might not have been as lonely as I thought.

There can be other causes for guilt as well. Children and teenagers who want to go out and spend time with their friends or who develop romantic relationships after the loss of a parent may feel that they are being disloyal—and in some families, they may even be told this.

It is difficult for teenagers to negotiate the complex and dichotomous feelings after a loss. The desire to go on with life and to be with others who are not sad contrasts with the pull to take care of other loved ones who are still grieving. The desire to have some fun contrasts with the undertow of sadness and remembering.

Ironically, guilty feelings may also play a positive role in the grief process. If a child or teen feels they caused the loss, they feel some power over what has happened. They feel a sense of potentially having been able to control an event that was actually uncontrollable. At times the fantasy of control, even when it leads to feelings of guilt and remorse, is preferable to the sense of having had no control at all.

And in regard to moving forward after loss, in most cases, the natural developmental process of maturation will motivate the child or adolescent toward forward movement. It will motivate them to do the things that they would normally be doing at their age—spending time with friends, going back to school, and resuming normal activities. At the very same time, children and teens who have suffered the loss of a parent may question whether these things are all right to do or whether they make any sense to do.

Another issue for children who have lost a parent is that their normal feelings of safety and security can be interfered with. Children and teenagers can develop a heightened fear of further loss. They may worry that their remaining parent will die, or they may have more concerns over loss in other relationships. Teens who develop intimate relationships may find themselves afraid of a breakup, they may become overly dependent on their partner, or—the opposite—they may resist getting too close to anyone. They may become overly independent and keep themselves out of intimate relationships in which dependency could occur.

Blending Families After the Death of a Parent

Eventually, a parent who has lost their partner may want to find someone with whom to have a new relationship. And once the parent finds someone they feel they would like to continue seeing, they may consider introducing this new partner to their children. If you are in this position, you may wonder what effect doing so will have on your children.

For example, Matt, whose story I tell in chapter 6, came to see me several months after his wife's death due to a prolonged illness. He talked a great deal about his two children and wanted my assistance in helping them deal with their mother's death. After spending almost the entire first session talking about this, I asked him how he was doing with his own mourning process.

He was initially reluctant to say too much, but he did tell me that he was very lonely and that he felt unprepared to do the job of both mother and father for his children.

Over the months, I would ask him more or less the same question at the end of each of our sessions—to the point that it became a running joke. He knew that he was reluctant to talk about himself and he knew that I knew this too—but that I would keep pushing him a little bit more each time to do so.

Gradually, he began to wonder if it would be all right to start to date. He wondered how his children would feel—and, in fact, how he himself would feel.

After about two years he began to talk about actually going on some dates. He was still sad, he still missed his wife terribly, and at the same time he felt that he needed to do more for himself. He was not sure how proceed or if this was the right thing for his children.

It took some time for Matt to weigh his desire to do everything he could for his children to prevent them any further suffering against his own needs for adult companionship. And it also took time for him to work through his own intense loyalty toward his late wife and to begin to value his own need to move forward.

Some parents will try to manage this process on their own, some will rely on friends and family for help and advice, and some will use psychotherapy as a way to work on their path forward after loss.

Matt used our work together to find his way. He slowly began to date, and together we decided that his children really did not need to know very much about this process. We both felt it would be unnecessarily upsetting for them to think about their father dating when he did not even have any prospects for a serious relationship yet. When he went out, he left his children with their familiar babysitter, he stayed in the neighborhood, and he told his children that he was having dinner with a friend.

After another year and a half, a total of three and a half years after his wife's death, Matt finally found someone with whom he felt he could have a committed and loving relationship. But introducing this fact to his children was not easy. Both children had gotten used to having their father to themselves and bringing a new person into the picture was threatening. One child wondered if her father would still love her as much. The other felt strongly that his father was being disloyal to his mother and her memory.

Matt talked with his children each time a concern came up. He dealt with their fears and their feelings as best he could, using a combination of sensitivity and rational expectations for their behavior toward his girlfriend.

Finally, Matt and his new partner decided it was time to live together. By this time one child was off at college and the other was in high school. Again, this was not an easy transition. There were many tough moments, feelings were hurt, a large number of discussions were needed about how each person was feeling and why—but eventually this new, now blended family was able to settle into a livable arrangement.

As in this example, some children will react negatively to the introduction of a new adult into their lives. Some will feel even more angry than the two children I have described here. But in other cases, children, especially very young children, may welcome a new adult, particularly if that person is sensitive, kind, and thoughtful about their needs.

In all of these situations, understanding what it feels like from the child's or teen's point of view is of the utmost importance. This will help in the transition. To facilitate this, the original parent can talk to their child about the child's feelings. For example, the parent can start off a conversation by saying something like "I know it's hard to have my boyfriend come over. It makes you remember that Daddy isn't here. It might take you a long time to get used to the fact that Daddy isn't here, because it's just so sad."

Everyone, including both the parent and the new partner, needs to know that a lost parent can never be replaced. If a new boyfriend, girlfriend, or partner enters the picture, it is important for that person to manage their own expectations. As much as they might want to be, they are not going to be the new parent. They are going to be a new person in the child's or teen's life and the child or teen may or may not welcome them. The new partner needs to have a detailed understanding of what the child has been through and what they are currently feeling. They must try to respect these feelings, and they must prepare for many ups and downs as everyone adjusts to the new situation.

This is a transition that will take time as well as innumerable conversations. Combining households may have to take longer than the new partner or the bereaved parent would like. They may need to go more slowly and more carefully than they would choose if there were not children involved.

New partners can feel hurt or angry that the child involved does not welcome them. They may feel upset that the child's feelings are coming before their own. At times they may feel that they have taken on more than they bargained for. But it is important for them to understand that the children in the family also have strong feelings and are having to make compromises they are not happy with after the loss of their parent.

Continuing Connections

Mourning a parent who has died means that the child will, very gradually, give up some of their investment in the relationship with that parent in order to make room for new attachments. But at the same time, the child will also have a continuing connection with their lost parent that will last throughout their lifetime.

They will often develop an internalized representation of the parent as well as an internal relationship with their parent, which can be comforting and stabilizing. By this I mean that the lost parent will become a part of the child. The lost parent's voice may become part of the child's conscience, and this voice may define what the child understands as right and wrong. Some of the lost loved one's habits and characteristics may become part of the child's way of being.

The child will spend time thinking about what their parent might have said or thought or done in innumerable circumstances. They may imagine what their parent would have said or done or wanted as a guide for their own decision-making and behavior.

Inevitably the child will also judge herself using standards that she perceives as her parent's standards. She may be critical of herself when she does things that she thinks the parent would have disliked, and she may feel good about herself and better connected to her lost parent when she does things she imagines that her parent would have liked or approved of.

And another thing: children will re-mourn their parent as they reach new stages of development or attain various achievements in their life. At graduations or birthdays, wedding days or other occasions, the lost parent will be poignantly remembered and missed all over again.

This, in and of itself, is a form of connection.

Children and teens who lose a parent will want and need this connection. They may remember their parent on certain days, as mentioned above, and they may try to remember their parents at other times. In the absence of an ability to bring the parent sufficiently to mind they may develop a belief in their parent's imagined presence. The lost parent may even appear through mystical phenomenon and in dreams.

Séamas O'Reilly, whose mother died when he was five, poignantly described this in his memoir:

> I don't have many memories of my mother. I do know that I dreamt about her a lot after she died. And those dreams were of us in heaven. The dreams were all the same pretty much . . . she wouldn't be bathed in light or descending from the clouds. She would be normal, unheralded, domestic. In the dreams she was never just there. I had to find her . . . there was never a big fanfare, but rather a commonplace discovery . . . and anyway, she's doing something, a commonplace thing, mending a shirt or wetting a cloth to wipe away a smudge on a tiny trouser leg.[7]

Sometimes children find these dreams comforting. Other times, they revive the memory of their lost parent so vividly that it is jarring and sad to wake up and remember that the parent is no longer alive.

The loss of a parent is a devastating event for a child of any age. It is a loss like no other and one that will change who the child is and what their future looks like. It is a loss that is felt throughout the child's life, into adulthood and old age.

The Loss of a Sibling

The impact of the loss of a sibling cannot be overestimated. Like the loss or death of a parent, it upends a child's life. In fact, everything changes for a child when their brother or sister is lost.

And the loss of a sibling can take a number of forms. The loss can occur through death, but it can also be caused by changes in the family structure. The child who goes to live with one parent while her sibling goes to live with the other, or the child who is left at home when their sibling leaves, is often very upset by the separation and experiences this change as a true loss. The child will feel that their life has changed in a way that they did not expect, and they can feel extremely lonely and abandoned.

The loss of a sibling which occurs as a result of something other than death is a type of "ambiguous loss," which I will describe further in chapter 5.

For example, Marta was eight when her older sister left for college. She had heard all the talk about applying to colleges, about acceptances and rejections, and she had been there during the packing process, but she didn't fully recognize what it would mean to have her sister be gone for months at a time. The apartment felt emptier without her sister. And although she also had a twelve-year-old brother, he did not make up for the fact that her sister was no longer at home. Her brother was a pest, while her sister had treated her specially; her sister had done her hair for her in the mornings. She had also slammed the door in Marta's face when her friends were over, making Marta furious. But still, Marta missed her sister more than she imagined that she would. It seemed like forever until Christmas when her sister would come home for the holidays. Her daily life was emptier, lonelier, different.

It is far worse when a sibling dies. This is a special kind of child-hood loss that deserves particular attention.

No loss in childhood, aside from the loss of a parent, comes as such a shock or subjects a child to as much suffering and foreclosed possibil-ities as the loss of a brother or sister. The loss of a sibling brings death too close. Children who lose a sibling have to confront death in a way that challenges all their beliefs about their own safety and mortality.

There is a new awareness that it is not just old people who die. The child is forced to realize that they themselves or any of their friends or other relatives could die at any time.

And there are other meanings—suddenly a member of the child's world is gone, an entire relationship ceases to exist in the real world, a whole piece of the child's life goes with the sibling who has died. Every day will be different from now on. The playing, the teasing, the fights, the hugs with that sibling—all gone.

The child who loses a brother or sister has opportunities at almost every point in the day to miss that sibling. And the child's whole future is changed as well. A relationship that would have existed through adulthood is gone. All family occasions will be different now.

In *The Empty Room: Understanding Sibling Loss*, Elizabeth DeVita-Raeburn writes about the aftermath of the death of her older brother as she watches his casket lowered into the ground at his funeral: "[I'm] not ready. . . . I feel numb, incredulous. . . . I don't want to go on, brother-less. I don't know how."[8]

It is hard to understand death at any age. But for a child to under-stand death is even harder. Where did the person who was just here go? How can they be gone?

This feeling of incredulousness is universal. And it is especially strong for children who have had little experience with death or who had little preparation for this particular death.

Sibling relationships are important—and they are complicated. They play an important role in who the child feels herself to be. They play an enormous part in a child's experience of daily life, and they help a child learn how to get along with other people. A sibling can be so many things—an adversary, a playmate, a role model, an example of what *not* to be like.

Siblings struggle over who gets to play with which toy, and they vie for parental attention. As they get older, they may compete academically, in sports, when playing board games or computer games, and in innumerable important—and silly—ways. Siblings fight, wrestle, pester, tease, and sometimes hate each other. And during a fight or in moments of anger, it is normal for children to wish their siblings gone. So, if a sibling actually dies, the surviving children may feel guilty for any of their hateful feelings or any aggression that was directed at the sibling.

They also share, cooperate, negotiate, coexist, comfort, protect, and love one another—and in experiencing all these feelings and behaviors, siblings learn how to negotiate relationships with others.

Children frequently define themselves in relation to their siblings. You will often hear a child say, "My brother is the smart one. I'm good at sports." Or "My sister is the pretty one." Often it seems that there can only be one of each kind in a family—as if all the children can't be smart or pretty at the same time. But inevitably children compare themselves to their siblings and put themselves in a particular place in the pecking order in regard to their siblings.

And each sibling relationship is unique. Even within a family, any parent who has more than two children knows that each sibling relates to another sibling differently. And these relationships can change from moment to moment, year to year.

The loss of a sibling changes everything. The dynamics of the family change. A child who was one of two becomes an only child. A child who was the middle child becomes the oldest. Or the youngest.

All future family experiences will be different than they would have been.

In *The Empty Room*, DeVita-Raeburn wrote about her experience of being the sister of "the boy in the bubble." Ben had an autoimmune disease that made him vulnerable to every germ and virus. As a result, he lived in a "bubble" at the National Institutes of Health for eight years—until he died at age eighteen.

DeVita-Raeburn said that after his death, "What I really wanted was to be happy, to be normal. But I didn't know how to make that happen." Her life, her daily reality, had been so shaped by her brother's illness and treatment that once he was gone, she did not know what to do with her own life. "Though I craved normalcy, I was much more comfortable with stress and crisis. I found everyday sameness—breakfast, lunch, dinner . . . unnerving. I struggled with the most mundane tasks."[9]

She wrote about feeling estranged from others, at times trying to make herself invisible. And after she met someone else who had lost a sibling during childhood, she wrote, "I had thought I was the only one. I thought losing a sibling was my own strange story."

She also tells how rare it was for anyone to ask about her experience. So often people asked about how her parents were and failed to ask about how she was doing and what it was like for her to have lost her only sibling. She described feeling that her brother's loss was not hers to mourn—it was her parents'. She was told explicitly and implicitly that "they" were having a hard time, and she should be a good child and not give them anything more to worry about. She said that everyone seemed to understand her parents' loss—but no one seemed to understand hers.

DeVita-Raeburn makes so many important points in her book. She talks about how difficult the loss of a sibling is for those children who loved their brother or sister but also for those who had a troubled relationship with their sibling. She both loved her brother and had a complicated relationship with him.

She described the loss of her brother in painful detail. She was fourteen when he died, and she was with him at the hospital when it happened. She talked about how surreal it felt in the hours leading up to his death and how shocked she felt after he died. She talked about her guilt at being able to sleep the night after he died, the sadness of returning to a house he would never again inhabit, and the pain of outliving him.

She also talked about how her parents' preoccupation after he died made her feel as if the wrong sibling had lived—she felt that her parents loved her brother more and that there was no way she could ever be loved as much as he had been. This is a common fantasy among children who lose a sibling. Not only do they have to be "good" to help their parents after the death, but at the same time, they often feel that they can never be good enough to make their parents happy again. All of this is part of the loss of a sibling.

Continuing Connections

The sibling relationship is more important than we often give it credit for. Our brothers and sisters help to shape who we are. If they are older, we use them as examples of how to be. We often idealize them and their abilities and yearn to be like them. In doing so, we find motivation to perform, to try harder, to achieve more. Depending on the family atmosphere, we also feel all sorts of feelings including jealous and competitive feelings. Likewise, if they are younger, we often feel superior, we may enjoy bossing them, and we may also learn how to care for them, protect them, and feel empathic toward them.

When a sibling is lost, our role as older or younger sibling to that child is gone. Our relationship with them is gone, an entire piece of our life is completely gone. And that may feel unbearable.

To acknowledge that a sibling is gone forever and that the relationship with them is completely over may be so intolerable that the child who has lost a sibling to death will continue to have a relationship with that sibling. They will continue to miss and to love their dead sibling. They will even continue to idealize that sibling, to compete with them or feel jealous of them—or any of the other feelings they had toward them during their time together.

And this will go on throughout their childhood and adolescence and into adulthood. They may imagine what their sibling might think about various issues, what opinions they might have, what they might say or think about what is going on in the family. The sibling will be a continuing presence in the inner life of the child and the child may imagine an eventual reunion in heaven.

They may also take on certain characteristics of the sibling who has died, they may take on some of their roles in the family, and they may feel that for their parents' sakes, they need to replace this sibling in the family. And this is part of their continuing connection to their sibling.

The Loss of a Grandparent

While it is the normal order of things for a grandparent to die during the life of a child, such an event can be a salient moment. If a child and their grandparent were close, it is, of course, an extremely sad and painful experience. A grandparent can be a unique source of love, comfort, and support for a child. Grandparents often do not have to discipline as much as parents. They can indulge the child's wants and needs more than the parents, and as such, the child may feel particularly upset when a grandparent dies, a sad emptiness where once there was a special kind of love and security.

Additionally, the loss of a grandparent may be the first death a child experiences up close. This is sometimes the first introduction to the concept of death as a real entity in the here and now for a child.

As I mentioned when I talked about the feelings a child can have after the death of a sibling, after a grandparent dies, the child can have all new fears about death, and it may occur to them that their own mother or father could die or even that they themselves could die.

This can raise existential issues for the child. What is death? What does it mean to die? These questions are difficult and parents may struggle to answer them.

But unlike when a sibling dies, with the death of a grandparent the discussion can include ideas about what it means to lead a long and productive life. It can be comforting for the child to know that the grandparent was older and got to have many years of life.

When explaining why the grandparent died, simple answers are best for younger children, based on the family's spiritual and religious beliefs. For older children, the conversation can be more nuanced, with parents asking their children what they think and believe as well as providing answers based on their own beliefs.

There can also be a double loss when a grandparent dies. The child not only feels her own feelings of loss but she must also deal with the grief of her parent who has lost a parent. It may be a new and troubling experience to see a parent cry or to be sad for an extended period of time—and that parent may be less available for a while, both emotionally and in terms of doing all the things they usually do for the child.

For example, Kyra was six when her grandmother died. They had not had a particularly close relationship as her grandmother had lived in another city and also because her grandmother was rather aloof as a person. But still, Kyra had questions. She asked her mother what happens after death. When her mother answered, "Nothing," Kyra became preoccupied by the idea of "nothing." What could it be like to be dead and be "nothing"? Where *was* her grandmother and what was it like for her? And what would happen when Kyra herself became "nothing"? Kyra didn't speak to anyone about her worries, but she found herself thinking about being "nothing" every night while trying to fall asleep.

Or, for another example, Jacob was twelve when his grandfather died. Jacob loved his grandfather dearly and had seen him often during his first eleven years of life. He did all he could to help his grandfather in the last months of his grandfather's life, visiting often, cleaning up his grandfather's yard, and bringing him his favorite bagels.

Jacob was alarmed as his grandfather's appearance began to change. His grandfather became more and more pale, and he was thinner each time Jacob saw him. After visits, Jacob would go to his room and take a nap. Clearly, being with his grandfather was something he wanted, but it was also disturbing and depleting for him.

Jacob's parents were worried about him and asked a friend who was a therapist whether or not Jacob should continue to visit his grandfather as frequently. The friend suggested that Jacob come to see him, and he took the time to sit down with Jacob to talk with him about his grandfather. Knowing that Jacob was interested in science, the friend thought that it might help to explain what was happening inside his grandfather's body. They talked about aging and why certain organs begin to break down. And they talked about how hard it is to watch as this happens to someone you love.

Jacob left the friend's house in a lighter mood. Because he was a boy who used his intellect to help him understand and process things, he had benefited from learning more about why his grandfather was losing weight and what the future might look like.

He continued to visit his grandfather often, and while very sad after each visit, he seemed more able to manage his sadness than he had been previously.

Continuing Connections

There are so many ways that a child can feel a continued connection to a grandparent. Often they cherish memories of things they did together. Or they replay advice their grandparent gave them. Some love to hear funny or interesting stories about their grandparent, and some will love to have something that belonged to their grandparent.

Some children may want to visit the cemetery where their grandparent is buried; some may want to bring flowers or a stone to put at the grave. Some may want to attend religious remembrances, and some may want to do none of these things.

In all cases, even if the relationship with the grandparent was not entirely positive, it is important for the adults in the family to bring up that grandparent in conversation from time to time so that the child knows that when someone has died, they are not forgotten and that we can continue to think about our lost loved ones and to process what they meant to us throughout our lives.

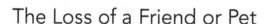

The Loss of a Friend or Pet

Friends are of the utmost importance to children. Throughout childhood, friends learn how to compete, cooperate, play, fight, and make up. Friends are the yardsticks against whom children measure themselves. With their friends, children can be themselves and learn who they are.

If a friend moves away, changes schools, becomes ill, or dies, this can be a grievous loss for the child.

Children depend on their friends—whether for after-school entertainment or for a feeling of security while at school. Friends can serve as buffers from what would otherwise feel like a threatening and anxiety-provoking experience, such as the first day of school, any given day in the cafeteria, or an experience with a bully. Friends can commiserate around a bad grade or a bad day. They can gossip together, form an alliance against other children, or go together to new activities which might otherwise be too scary to join.

If a close friend, and especially a best friend, is no longer there to provide company or comfort or commiseration, the child can suddenly feel quite insecure. They can miss their friend, feel anxious without their friend, or worry whether they will ever be able to make another good friend. As many parents know, if a good friend is even absent from school for a few days, this can be a difficult thing for the child. Sometimes, a child can feel quite lost when their best friend is not there to sit next to at lunch or play with at recess. This too is an "ambiguous loss"—not a permanent loss, but one that requires acknowledgement nonetheless (chapter 5, page 116).

The same is true with the loss of a beloved pet. Pets can provide a truly intimate relationship for a child. Sometimes the child can feel that their pet is the only being who truly understands them or with whom they can genuinely be themselves. Often, a pet provides a safe haven for a child. Pets offer love and affection without judgment and give the child someone to care for without the complications of human relationships. When a pet dies, the child will need time to be sad, to contemplate and process what death means, and to be angry about the unfairness of death.

The child who has lost a pet may appreciate being able to hold a little funeral for the pet, and they are often best off having some time to process their loss before acquiring a new pet.

While some children will ask for a new pet right away, or some parents might offer to provide a new pet immediately, in either case, this is an attempt to avoid the pain of loss—for the child or for the adults witnessing the child's pain—and it is not the best solution. It is important for the adults in the child's life to convey the message that loss is hard, but that we can sit with our sad feelings, we can feel them, and we can survive them.

Continuing Connections

Children may have a continuing connection with a special friend who has moved or died. They may continue to miss the friend, and think and perhaps talk about their friend for a long time.

Parents are well advised to ask how the child is feeling both immediately after the loss and in the ensuing weeks and months. While a parent might hope that the child will get "over" the loss quickly and move on to other friends, this is often not the case. Even if the child does make other friends, that does not mean that the lost friend is any less important to them on an ongoing basis.

Children may also have a continued connection with a special pet who has died. They may look at photos of the pet, hold on to the collar, keep a tuft of fur, or insist on not getting rid of something that the pet cherished. They may replay the funeral with their stuffed animals, or talk about the pet and ask questions about their death for days or weeks or months to come.

The loss of a parent, sibling, grandparent, friend, or pet is an extremely significant event in a child's life. While the death of a parent is undoubtedly the most difficult and painful loss, all of these losses will shape the child and her perception of herself, her life, and, in the case of a death, her ideas about mortality and her own mortality in particular.

In the following chapter, I will talk about how the manner of loss, in part, determines the child's reaction to the loss and how she is affected by it. I will talk about divorce, illness, violence, war, and suicide and how each of these can affect children.

CHAPTER 4

Different Manners of Loss

We've explored how children and teens grieve and mourn at different ages, and how they might feel and react when a loved one disappears from their lives. In this chapter, we will look at various manners of loss, including divorce, illness, violence, war, and suicide.

Apart from death, there are other ways to lose someone, which we need to consider. The losses that occur through divorce or illness must also be mourned. When a parent who was present seven days a week is only available for two or three days per week due to a custody arrangement following divorce, this is a huge loss for a child. Daily life and family routines change completely. And the relationship with each parent changes. These differences need to be acknowledged and any sadness or anger around them needs to be expressed and processed. When a parent becomes ill, this is another immense loss. Often the parent can no longer do all of the things they did before they became ill. In some ways they may no longer be the person they were before. This must be acknowledged to help the child process the significance of their parent's illness for them.

And there are particular ways of losing a loved one to death that require specific attention, including through violence, war, or suicide. All of these are complicated, and I will talk at length about each.

Loss Due to Divorce

When a child's parents divorce, their entire world changes.

The emotional environment of the home may be full of conflict before, during, or after a divorce happens. One or both parents may be very upset, angry, sad or depressed. There may be talk of lawyers, courtrooms, and money. Life is a roller coaster of uncertainty for quite a while.

And in so many ways, the child will never again have what she had before. Her nuclear family, as a unit, has been destroyed. The child's living situation changes, with whom she lives changes, new stepparents and new stepsiblings or half-siblings may enter the picture.

Meanwhile, the parents' experience of the divorce and its aftermath may be completely different than it is for their children.

When Kevin was twelve, his parents divorced. After his father moved out, Kevin felt a new sense of vulnerability. Suddenly he was afraid of break-ins in a way that he had not been when his father lived at home. He felt less protected and less safe than he ever had before. He also felt that he had to be responsible for his two siblings. He cooked them breakfast on the weekends while his mother slept late, and he tried to take care of them emotionally when they were scared or felt lonely. He also wanted to take care of his mother now that she did not have a husband. He helped out more around the house and he refrained from complaining too much about things so that she wouldn't have to worry that he wasn't happy.

When his mother went out at night and he and his siblings spent time with a babysitter, he missed his mother terribly and he worried about her. He was frightened on those nights—and until his mother returned home he wondered if she would come home at all. He worried she would get into a traffic accident and he worried that she might die. Then, when his mother married again a year later, he found himself living with a new stepfather he did not particularly like.

When his parents divorced, Kevin lost the daily relationship with his father. He only saw his father every other weekend and one night during the week for dinner. It felt strange and lonely at mealtimes when he was with his mother and his father was not at the table. He missed being able to go to his father for help with homework. He lost the sense of safety and security he had previously felt when his father was in the house. He took on some of the jobs his father did around the house, but his mother had to take on the rest. She became cranky and easily irritated. She spoke angrily about Kevin's father, and this put Kevin in a terrible situation because he still loved his father. Kevin didn't know whether to believe the things his mother said or whether to be loyal to his father and fight back when his mother said these things. Kevin's mother also had to move with him and his brother to several different apartments, so he also lost his original home and neighborhood. But more than any of that, Kevin lost his ability to just be the child he had been before the divorce—a more secure and care-free version of himself.

Meanwhile, Kevin's parents had very little idea of how he was feel-ing. Kevin's father was deeply depressed and was not able to function very well day to day. He was lost in his own world of misery and had very little capacity to reflect on what Kevin might be going through.

Kevin's mother was also depressed—and angry—and she was mostly just concentrating on how to survive. She relied on Kevin to be of help and, like his father, she had very little bandwidth for considering what Kevin was feeling and what effect all this might be having on him.

Kevin, like many children whose parents divorce, really lost both parents—at least as they had been when they were together. The only way Kevin could figure out how to respond was to become the helper for each parent. He tried to take on some of his father's roles with his mother, a situation that was emotionally quite difficult for him. And he tried to rouse his father from his depression by urging him to clean up his apartment and by suggesting places they could go and things they could do on the weekends.

Kevin had to mature beyond his years as a result of his parent's divorce. He reacted to the divorce by trying his best to get each of his parents back to normal. This altered his development and shaped his personality, causing him to mature prematurely and to take on the helper role as part of his identity.

There is usually a great deal of upset during and after a divorce. And as it turns out, even worse than the initial confusion caused by the announcement of a divorce and the consequent reshuffling of liv-ing arrangements is the conflict between the parents witnessed by the children in the family. Both before and after divorce, conflict between the parents has been shown to be the most harmful and upsetting aspect of divorce for children. Any arguing, fighting, or ill will between parents is excruciating for the child, as they usually love both people and do not want to see either one hurt.

When there is heightened conflict between the parents, children are overexposed to anger and aggression. This is frightening for children no matter their age. And they can feel quite confused. After all, each parent is part of them. They are genetically related to both their mother and their father, and they undoubtedly share physical characteristics, personality traits, habits, likes and dislikes with them. So if the mother criticizes the father, what does this mean about the child? What does this mean about the part of them that is genetically like the father? What does this mean about the personality or physical characteristics they share with the father? Does this mean that the mother no longer loves this part of them?

Many children of parents who have been in conflict remember overhearing their parents arguing and feeling scared and helpless. Some children try to intervene on behalf of one parent or the other. Others run and hide. Some try to protect their siblings and to shield them from conflict or violence. Some children have had to call the police—and some have lived their lives regretting that they did not call the police. These memories last into adulthood, and these events have long-lasting effects on the children involved, on their development, on their sense of self, and on their future relationships.

Loss Due to Illness

Another type of loss occurs when a loved one is ill. Whether the loved one is temporarily ill or ill from a condition that will not improve, the situation is complicated. The confusing aspect of this situation involves the fact that when someone is ill, they are still alive, and they are available in some ways. However, they may be much less available than they were when they were well—and for children, as well as for the rest of us, this loss is difficult to deal with and difficult to talk about.

We are often so preoccupied with worrying about the ill person and figuring out how to get them the best care that we fail to acknowledge what we have lost. Is our ill loved one unable to do all the activities they used to do with us? Are they unable to communicate well or to remember us? Are they less able to give and express love? Are they more preoccupied?

For children, these losses matter. Am I allowed to be sad that Mommy is sick and can't pick me up and carry me anymore? Or do I have to just be nice and try to help her all the time? Am I allowed to be angry that Grandpa didn't remember my name? Or do I have to pretend that didn't happen? Am I allowed to complain that Daddy can't go outside and play? Or should I just be quiet and go out and play by myself? Who do I talk to about feeling confused when my mother doesn't get up out of bed when I need her?

A father, Samuel, told me that his wife had had a sudden stroke and was in a rehabilitation hospital following many days in the hospital. He had told his four-year-old daughter, Lily, that Mommy was sick and that the doctors were trying to help her, but Lily was missing her more and more, having trouble going to sleep at night and generally being more irritable during the day.

Samuel was at his wit's end. He had a four-month-old baby, a four-year-old, and a wife who was in the rehabilitation hospital with an uncertain future. He was fairly sure that what he had told his daughter so far was the right thing—but it was not "working."

To help this young father, I had to think with him about what must have been in his daughter's mind. I suggested that we think like a four-year-old, and together we started to understand how confusing it must be for Lily. Mommy was still not at home. Why was she gone so long? Lily's understanding of being sick was based on her own experience of having a cold for a few days and staying home from preschool.

I helped Samuel to be able to talk to his little girl about how frustrating it was that Mommy wasn't coming home and to acknowledge how much they *both* missed her. I also suggested that he be honest with Lily and tell her that the doctors did not know when Mommy would be able to come home, even though they were trying their best to help her.

Then the question came up as to whether Lily should go see her mother. The mother was unable to walk on her own, and her cognitive abilities and capacity for speech had not completely returned. If she had visitors, she would be in a wheelchair pushed by an aide.

What would this be like for Lily? Would it be better for her to see her mother or would it be more confusing?

Embedded in her mother's illness were many ambiguous losses for this little girl. Her mother was still alive, but she was not at home. She still existed somewhere in the world, but Lily didn't understand exactly where she was or why she was there.

Lily had lost her mommy in her everyday life, she had lost the time she spent with her mommy, and she had lost all the love and care her mother provided for her. And if she went to see her mother? She would lose her image of her mother as a big, strong mommy. She would see her looking ill and unable to walk or talk well.

Similarly, if a grandparent is suffering from dementia or Alzheimer's disease, the child may feel confused. She may think, Grandpa is still here, but he doesn't remember the song we used to sing, he doesn't ask me how school is anymore, or, even worse, he doesn't remember *me*.

Illness can be a loss that is more complicated even than a loss due to death. Often there is no quick resolution—a parent or grandparent may be ill for months or even years, leaving the children in the family with difficult absences in their lives. I will discuss this further in chapter 5.

In addition, when a parent or very close relative is ill, especially if they are terminally ill, there will usually be a sense of crisis in the family. The constant stress and worry will affect every member of the family, especially the children. The sense of a progressively worsening situation will feel burdensome to the children, and they, like other family members, may develop a fear of the inevitable death of their loved one.[1]

To help the children in the family, it is important to keep them updated in real time about the progress of the illness. Explain what is happening as it is happening. This is crucial because without information, the child cannot prepare herself for what is to come. If the parent or close relative is going to get worse or if they are going to die eventually, the child needs to be able to anticipate this and to have all her feelings about it. Without such preparation, her mourning may be more complicated and more difficult to progress through later.[2]

Also, it is important to remember that when a family member is ill, toddlers and young children may feel overwhelmed by their parent's dramatic feelings. Grace Hyslop Christ tells a story in her book *Helping the Grieving Child* about Rachel, a two-and-a-half-year-old whose father had leukemia and whose health was failing. When Rachel and her mother entered the hospital room to visit Rachel's father, Rachel's mother started crying, her father started crying, and they all hugged. The next day when Rachel went to the hospital with her mother, she did not want to enter her father's room and she seemed angry with her father. Her mother realized that Rachel had been overwhelmed by her parents' strong emotions and that she and her husband had to keep their most intense grief separate from their interactions with Rachel.[3]

Similarly, a few months later, Rachel's mother came home from the hospital exhausted and upset. Rachel began to cry, and her mother began to cry at the same time. Rachel's mother thought they were having a good cry together, but the next day Rachel said, "Remember yesterday I was crying? You were crying too. I was crying first. Two people aren't allowed to cry at the same time."[4]

Toddlers and small children—and for that matter, children of any age—may worry when their parent becomes very upset. They worry that their parent won't be able to comfort or take care of them. And in fact, this is true. If a parent is overwhelmed by their own feelings, their caretaking ability will be diminished. So when one parent is quite ill, the other parent is in an extremely difficult situation. They have their own immense sadness and worry—and they have their responsibility to care for and reassure their children.

In such cases, the well parent will have to figure out if they can compartmentalize their own strong feelings and express them at times when they are with other adults or when they are by themselves. If not, they have to figure out how bring in other adults to care for their children, for at least some of the time, so that the children have calm, emotionally available adults to comfort them and answer their questions.

In Rachel's case, her mother realized that it was not helpful for Rachel to see her when she was extremely upset about her husband's condition. She talked to Rachel about how Rachel did not like her mother to cry when she was the one who started crying first, and she told Rachel that she would try not to do this in the future.

Loss Due to Violence

Part of what was so difficult for me about my father's death was that it happened suddenly and without warning. Weeks after he died, we discovered that my father had been suffering from coronary artery disease and chest pain for years, but he had kept this a secret. When my brother cleaned out my father's medicine cabinet, he found all sorts of medications that my father had been taking—without our knowledge.

Knowing that my father was ill would not have made losing him any easier, but it might have lessened the shock. Losing a beloved relative or friend is hard enough, but losing them with no preparation is even harder. Shock becomes part of the experience of loss.

And when loss occurs due to violence, it is not only sudden, it is not only shocking, it is undeniably traumatic and life-altering.

I wrote this chapter minutes after hearing about the mass shooting at Robb Elementary School in Uvalde, Texas. I do not have to hear any of the details of this particular tragedy to know that parents, children, staff, and the entire Uvalde community have been traumatized.

And it is not just Uvalde. There were 37 school shootings in the United States in 2023 that resulted in injuries or deaths, and as this book goes to press, there have been 181 such shootings since 2018 in the US.[5]

In each and every case, there has been horrific loss. Parents have lost children, children have lost parents, siblings have lost siblings, children have lost teachers, teachers have lost students, and everyone involved has lost any sense of safety and security that they might previously have had.

Proximity to violence is a loss unto itself.

Like living through a pandemic, those who have experienced violence or have been close to a violent event are robbed of their sense of trust in the world, and their trust in other human beings. They are often haunted by the event itself, and many times they have no idea how to cope with the experience or the feelings and the memories of the event, which may be frequent and intrusive.

The children and staff who were present at the shooting in Uvalde, the children and staff of the more general school community where the shooting occurred, the children in the community attending other schools, and, in fact, all the community members in general were affected and needed help following this event and others like it.

Many adults and children will suffer aftereffects, including fear of leaving home or going to school. They may also suffer from a more general feeling of anxiety. They might have intrusive memories, trouble concentrating, trouble sleeping, trouble calming themselves down—in fact, all the symptoms of posttraumatic stress disorder.

They will need frequent reassurance and comforting, they will need help going back to normal daily life, and they may need professional help. They will also need information to help them to understand what effect the experience of violence generally has on people.

At the same time, many people, including children and teens, find ways to channel their horror and loss into productive activities. We can think about some of the students from Marjory Stoneman Douglas High School in Parkland, Florida, where a mass shooting took place in 2018.

X (formerly Emma) González is perhaps the most well-known of these students. Almost immediately after the shooting, she leaped into action, speaking publicly about what happened at her school and advocating for new gun control laws. She is famous for saying, "We call B. S. on the lack of gun control action taken by politicians who are funded by the National Rifle Association." She is someone who turned her grief and anger into a productive form of outrage.[6]

While we do not know very much about González's inner life and in what ways she may still be suffering, we do know that, in general, it can be very helpful for children and teens to find a way to be active in their grief rather than feeling like a passive victim who can do nothing.

And then there is Eden Hebron, who was also a student at Marjory Stoneman Douglas, who watched as her best friend and two other classmates were shot.[7] For a while following the shooting, Eden kept going on with her life as usual, getting straight As and attending high school sports events with her friends. But eventually her family noticed that she was more argumentative than she had ever been, she was suspicious, sometimes even paranoid. She told others that she often felt scared and sad. And when she was alone, she cried.

Eden started drinking and went through a series of difficult relationships. She closed herself off from her parents while simultaneously presenting herself as a normal teenager when she went to school each day.

But Eden was anything but normal. She was traumatized and bereaved.

She acted out by drinking and getting involved in destructive relationships. So many feelings lay within her, unprocessed and unexpressed, and she did not know how to deal with them.

Her drinking was likely a form of self-medication—a way that she found to stop herself from thinking about the shootings, a way to

numb her pain and quiet her anxiety. The acting out, the various relationships she entered into, may have served a similar purpose. When
trauma and loss coincide, processing one may interfere with moving
through the grief for the other.

Grieving may be interfered with by the reaction to the trauma.

The anxiety and fear that come from being so close to death may
distract the child or teen from being able to feel sad about the loss of
loved ones. And the grief and mourning may interfere with the processing of all the complicated feelings that arise after having been
involved in a violent event or being close to one.

This is a complex journey and there is no roadmap for this trip—
no guaranteed way for a child or teen to navigate this experience.

Fortunately for Eden, her parents had the resources to find and
enroll her in a high-quality therapeutic treatment program in California. They were able to fly to California to visit her every other week
and eventually to move to California to be near her.

Once out of the program and living in the group home where she
went afterward, Eden continued psychotherapy, finished high school,
and moved on to college. At the time she was interviewed she said that
she recognized that her recovery was not complete and that she still
had to concentrate on taking care of herself.

Although several years have passed since the shooting, it is undoubt-
able that Eden and the other students who were at Stoneman Douglas
that day, and especially those who witnessed the shootings or lost friends,
are still processing their experiences and will be affected by them
throughout their lives, including as they become parents themselves.

Studies have been done on such teens. It has been shown that
among the issues that have arisen for them as they have become parents
are anxiety about the safety of their own children, struggles around
how to tell their children about their experience with violence, and
difficulty figuring out how to just live in a world where they know this
sort of violence can directly affect them or their children at any time.

One such survivor, Brenda Valenzuela, was profiled in an article
in the *New York Times*.[8] Brenda survived a community college

shooting during which she watched as her teacher and nine other students were shot. She had stepped outside the classroom to take a call on her cell phone and was able to see what was going on through the window of the classroom door.

Now, eight years later, she becomes extremely anxious about the safety of her two children at the beginning of each new school year. She makes sure they have the most bulletproof backpacks available, and she tracks their whereabouts on her phone throughout the school day. She is intensely anxious around the anniversary date of the shooting each year, and she can have panic attacks when she least expects it. Valenzuela has sought help and she feels she has tried everything, including medication, therapy, meditation, and a therapy dog, but she still suffers, especially when having to send her children to school.

There are many kinds of violence besides school shootings that can affect children and result in loss for them.

In my practice, I have seen a number of children who have experienced the loss of a parent by murder, sometimes perpetrated by the other parent. I have seen children who have been present as their homes were robbed (in one case, their Christmas tree and all their presents were taken). And I have seen children who have been in automobile or other kinds of accidents where a family member has died. All of these children have needed professional help, often over the course of years, in order to acknowledge, express, and work through their feelings. And their families have needed help learning how to support their children's recovery. But even with professional help, sadly, the effects of exposure to violence can be long term and even lifelong for both the child and the child's family.

Loss Due to War

Up until this point, I have discussed the consequences for children who have experienced one loss or who have been present at one violent event. But children who have lived—or are living—through war are in a separate category altogether. Often, they have suffered losses too numerous to count—including the loss of innocence, the loss of safety, and the loss of a sense of any kind of security, not to mention the actual losses of family, friends, teachers, community members, homes, schools, and entire neighborhoods.

As I write, children are dying and losing loved ones every single day in multiple locations around the globe, including all the wars referred to on page 4. These children are suffering in ways that are quite simply horrific and completely incompatible with normal development.

Globally, one in four children, or over 1.6 billion children worldwide live in a country affected by armed conflict, terrorism, or disaster.[9] And armed conflict can last throughout a child's entire life, such as in Liberia where civil war caused widespread trauma from 1989 to 2004.[10]

The effects of war are innumerable. They extend far beyond the trauma that is experienced by witnessing and being the victim of violence. They include the loss of home and community due to fighting and bombardment. They include evacuation and immigration and all the losses embedded in those experiences.

In 2016 alone, the United Nations High Commission on Refugees reported that 59.5 million people worldwide were forcibly displaced, and over half of these were children under the age of 18.[11] And we must remember that the numbers are even larger than this because there are many kinds of war—including not only armed conflicts between nations but also drug wars, gang wars, and more localized street fighting caused by conditions of poverty and social inequality.

The past two decades have marked increasing interest in the psychological impact of war on children. Many researchers have studied this subject, and the relationship between exposure to adverse childhood events, including war trauma, and the development of acute stress disorder, posttraumatic stress disorder (PTSD) and physiological and mental illness has been well documented.

We know that living in or near a war zone usually involves suffering multiple losses of all sorts over long periods of time. War often involves kidnapping, surprise attacks, sexual assault, forced family separation, enrollment of one or more family members in the military, and, most of all, the loss of family members and friends to death or displacement.

Children who live in war zones are often so traumatized that we are surprised when any of them manage to live through the experience and remain psychologically intact.

We know that in many cases having lived through war impacts the life trajectory of children far more than that of adults. Children who live through war often lose the opportunity for education, adequate health care, and normal social lives. Some children are forced to become child soldiers, some have to move into refugee or displaced person camps where they may wait for years in miserable circumstances for normal life to resume, if it ever does. Some may be injured or disabled in war, and as a result of these injuries they may be further deprived of opportunities even when the war is over.

As far as psychological effects of war on children are concerned, studies have shown that the severity, nature, and duration of the violence and trauma experienced by children are the best indicators of their level of later psychopathology and possibility for adaptation.[12]

However, it is also true that experiencing violence or terror can affect one child in one way and other child differently. One child may weather such events with few aftereffects while another may be deeply traumatized. And studies only go so far. They look for general trends. What happens to specific children cannot be adequately described by statistical or scientific studies. The immense tragedy of each child's losses cannot be measured.

Psychologists, psychiatrists, and public health researchers are only just beginning to understand what exacerbates the effect of trauma in one child and what protects another. When traumatic exposure has lasting effects on a child, it has been found that individual differences affect the degree to which the child does or does not recover.

The child's age and developmental stage at the time of the exposure to war and all the associated trauma affect her reaction. The youngest of children are often protected from the devastating effects of violence and war if they are able to stay with their mothers and if the mothers are able to be comforting and emotionally available during frightening events. Older children who are more aware of what is going on around them and who may witness acts of violence are more likely to be deeply affected.

Children who are psychologically healthy, who are flexible, well organized, and adaptable, are more likely to do better even under very difficult circumstances. On the other hand, children who are highly sensitive or who are neurodivergent (whether they are on the autistic spectrum, suffer from learning disabilities, physical illnesses, ADD or ADHD, and the like) are more likely to be adversely affected by the chaos and violence of war. But under extremely adverse conditions, even the healthiest and best put together of children will suffer tremendously.

In a short documentary called *What Is War to a Grieving Child?*, Mona El-Naggar, Jonah M. Kessel, and Alexander Stockton share the accounts of children in Ukraine who have lost their father in the war with Russia.[13]

This is what the children say:

"War is evil. War is death. It's a waste of time, a waste of everything. It's loss."

"I can't even go to my father's grave . . . I can't do it."

"I have such a hurricane in my soul."

"I even feel sorry for the Russian people. They have children who don't deserve to lose their dads."

One boy and his father were shot at point-blank range while riding their bikes. The boy survived by playing dead. His father did not.

Another teen said, "The war will end, but my father will not come back."

At the grief camp they attended, they were all asked to create dream houses. One made a Russian house, soaked in blood.

These kids didn't just lose their fathers—they lost their homes, pets, everything that made up their lives. One boy said, "After my father died, I began to appreciate things I'd never noticed. When he made tea and added sugar. Those sounds. I'll never be able to hear them again." A girl said, "I don't discuss anything at all with my mom. I thought if I showed any weakness it would be even worse for my mom."

It has also been shown that how parents react to difficult circumstances affects how children do. When mothers are less anxious or depressed, this is associated with better outcomes for children—and when fathers are less severely affected by their own PTSD, this is also associated with less PTSD in children.

The most common psychological problems for children who are living or who have lived through the conditions of war are worry, anxiety, separation anxiety, depression, PTSD, acting out, detachment, delinquency, bullying, drug and alcohol abuse, suicidal thoughts, and self-blame.[14]

Of course, most of these symptoms make sense. Children who have lived through war have been exposed to many, many scenes and experiences of terror and horror. They have seen things no one should have to see.

But the self-blame and suicidality? These require more explanation.

First of all, conditions of war have been shown to cause more abuse and violence within families. The fear, stress, and deprivation experienced in war can lead to hostile and violent acts even within the home against loved ones. These experiences, along with living through the violence of war itself, can stir up angry, hostile, and aggressive feelings within the child—both toward the family members who may have acted aggressively and toward the enemy.

We can feel anger and hatred toward anyone who has hurt us—whether these are people close to us or strangers who have invaded our country. And these feelings may lead to all sorts of fantasies of violent revenge. When children have such revenge fantasies, this can later lead to feelings of guilt and of having deserved whatever losses or injuries they suffered.

And suicidality? Well, the experience of extreme trauma, including violence and violent bereavement, can lead to feelings of hopelessness in some children. "What is the point of life?" is a question many children with these experiences will ask themselves. In some cases, such thoughts lead to thoughts of ending life. And feelings of anger and hatred can also lead to suicidal feelings. As Sigmund Freud formulated it, depression is anger turned inward—and to extend this formulation, suicidality can be a form of rage turned inward.

But there are also protective factors. As mentioned earlier, researchers from as long ago as World War II and as recently as 2022 have found that being cared for by parents during wartime can have a strong positive effect for children. This is especially true when these parents are able to remain loving toward their children.

One group of researchers[15] showed that, in a context of multiple traumas caused by war and natural disaster, parental care can moderate the severity of trauma experienced by children. It can also help children to develop fewer feelings of self-blame as well as fewer behavior problems. In this study, children who reported their parents to be highly caring did not show a significant increase in internalizing problems such as anxiety, depression, and social withdrawal related to their exposure to mass trauma.

Similarly, data from families in postwar Uganda revealed that the effect of war trauma on children was partially reduced by care from mothers and other female nurturers.[16] Likewise, during World War II, Anna Freud and Dorothy Burlingham found that the children who stayed with their mothers in London fared better than those sent to the countryside for their physical safety. Proximity to their mothers' love and care was a protection against the development of traumatic reactions, despite the fact that they lived in a city under almost constant bombardment.[17]

And it is also true that many children demonstrate incredible resilience.

Although war is horrific, especially for the children who must live through it, it is true that, amazingly, recovery is the expected outcome for most children who experience acute distress responses. This can give us just a bit of hope for those children who have been and who are currently being exposed to war.

Loss Due to Suicide

The idea that someone could kill themself on purpose is a horrifying idea for anyone, but especially for a child. And if a child loses someone to suicide, this will be especially shocking if the person did not show obvious signs of depression, disordered thinking, or a wish to die prior to killing themself.

The suicide of a loved one or a friend—or even of a well-known celebrity—raises all sorts of questions for children and teens: "Why would someone want to kill themself?" being the first and most profound of all. Answering this question requires a great deal of courage on the part of parents, teachers, and others who children may talk to about the subject.

This discussion must include explanations of depression, hopelessness, and mental and physical illness, topics which many adults are reluctant to bring up with children. Often adults prefer to believe that children and teens do not think too deeply about these matters, but the fact is that children and teens are actually very interested in these subjects—and in the most profound questions in life in general.

Of course, it is an especially sensitive matter when a parent or other very close relative dies by suicide. This is a devastating and life-altering event for a child or teen. And this is particularly so for children who witness the suicide or who find the parent after the suicide. This is a traumatic event of the highest magnitude.

An adult who was in psychotherapy remembered the terrible experience of finding his father when he was a young boy. He spoke of this to his analyst: "It was practically by chance that I went into the small room behind [my father's] office . . . in an instant the blue of my eyes became filled with the shape of Dad, who was hanging from the ceiling, A rope around his neck, a rope that left a blue mark on that crooked neck."[18]

What an absolutely horrible experience for this child, having to see his once strong, lively father now dead—and not only dead but having died in such a shocking and confusing way.

This young boy, like any child who experiences the death of a parent through suicide, was faced with the need to confront not only his parent's death but also the suddenness of the death, the shock of both the death and how it happened, the violence of the death, and the intentionality of the death.

As shown in this boy's description, a child who finds a parent who has died by suicide will be terrified, they will be sad, and they may be angry—all at the very same time. And this is why I call this experience traumatic. The child will be overwhelmed in all ways. In fact, all surviving members of a family in which someone has died by suicide are usually both shocked and traumatized. They often feel that the death was unnecessary, and it is common for them to blame themselves for the death.

Children in particular will often imagine that if only they had been more lovable or "better" kids, their parent or loved one would not have wanted to kill themself. They may wonder what they might have done differently in order to have prevented the suicide—and they may agonize over this question for a very long time.

Moreover, children and teenagers whose parent or close loved one dies by suicide will inevitably have a host of mixed feelings about the person who has died. Along with sadness and missing feelings, they may also feel furious that the person did this and/or guilty that they themselves were not able to prevent it.

To make matters worse, children whose parents have died by sui-cide are more at risk. First, they are more likely to have difficulty in the mourning process. Mourning will be complicated by their trau-matization and by their mixed feelings about the person who died. Second, they are more likely to experience thoughts about wanting to kill themselves. In one study,[19] it was found that children who had a parent who died by suicide were more than twice as likely as other children to have suicidal ideation and over six times as likely to have made a suicide attempt in the one-year period that was covered by the study.

These are serious numbers. Having a parent or close loved one die by suicide opens the door to suicide as a viable solution to hopelessness or depression. Children and teens who are depressed, angry, or dis-tressed in any one of many ways who have a family member who has killed themselves may see suicide as an acceptable strategy for dealing with their pain.

Divorce, illness, violence, war, and suicide are all events that con-tain multiple losses for children—and I have only just scratched the surface of the many negative effects each of these can have on the children who experience them.

Next, I will talk about a different sort of loss—the kind that is less obvious and less well defined.

CHAPTER 5

Ambiguous Loss

Ambiguous loss is "a loss that remains unresolved and unclear, without official verification or immediate resolution."[1] It is a type of loss in which it is not known if a loved one is dead or alive, absent or present.

It is different from most of the losses discussed so far.

It is the kind of loss that is life-altering—but not always recognized.

It is the kind of loss that is often not even thought about as loss.

It is the loss that we think of as part of everyday life, the loss that may not involve death, the loss that happens slowly, or the loss that occurs when something otherwise considered good is happening.

It can involve a loved one who is simply away for a prolonged period, such as a sibling who has gone to college or a mother who has been deployed by the military. It can involve a loved one who is injured or ill or missing, such as a grandparent who has broken her hip and is in rehab or an aunt who has early-onset Alzheimer's. It can even involve someone who is still present but who seems psychologically absent because they have taken on a new job, such as a mother who has received a promotion and now has to be at the office twelve hours a day, or because they are in mourning themselves, such as a father whose own father has died.

The term "ambiguous loss" was coined by Pauline Boss, a sociologist who grew up with a father who had emigrated from Switzerland. As a child, she noticed a pervasive sadness about her father, but she did not understand where it came from. She felt that her father was absent sometimes when he was actually present. Only later in her life did she realize that her father's sadness originated from having left his homeland and his family and that, as a sensitive child, she had picked up on his powerful missing feelings.

In the 1970s, Boss studied two types of families: one type being families in which the fathers were too busy working to take an active part in raising their children and the other type being the families of fighter pilots who were missing in action. In the first kind of family, she noted that the fathers were psychologically absent from their children's lives but physically present. In the other type of family, the fathers were psychologically present but physically absent. She saw that each type of family lived in a kind of limbo where their losses were not really named but where there was sorrow and grief anyway.

It is Pauline Boss who defined ambiguous loss as a situation of unclear loss in which it is not known if a loved one is dead or alive, absent or present.

She says, "Ambiguous loss is an extraordinary stressor—a producer of uncanny anxiety and unending stress that blocks coping and understanding. It freezes the grief process and defies resolution."[2]

Similar to ambiguous loss is "disenfranchised grief". Kenneth Doka formally introduced this term in 1989 and defined it as loss that is felt yet is not "openly acknowledged, socially validated, or publicly mourned."[3] He explained that sometimes those around us may not view our loss as significant, and they may think we don't have the right to grieve. They might not like how we may or may not be expressing our grief, and thus they may feel uncomfortable, or judgmental. He agreed with Boss that this sort of experience of grief might pose difficulties in terms of emotional processing and expression.

We can extend the term even further and use it to describe the experience of many of us over the time of the Covid-19 pandemic, just as Pauline Boss did in a later book.[4] Ambiguous loss was ubiquitous from 2020 to 2022. Even those who did not lose loved ones to illness lost other things during this time, including our normal way of life, our sense of safety, and our freedom to go where we pleased. And for the times of quarantine, we all lost our ability to be with friends and family, to go into school or offices, and to go about our daily lives as we had previously.

Even without a pandemic, ambiguous loss happens all the time. For example, ambiguous loss occurs when a teenager gets ready to go to college or into the military and then leaves. The teenager loses her childhood home and the proximity of her parents. The parents lose the everyday presence of their child. Siblings lose the presence of that sister or brother in the house.

Going to college is supposed to be a happy event! The teen has gotten into college and is going there to study and to learn how to be independent. But there are also many losses involved in this "happy" event.

Ambiguous loss also occurs as a sibling or parent prepares for military deployment and then goes off—or as couples decide to separate and then move into different apartments or houses.

No one has died, but a way of life has ended. The member of the military loses her home for the time being. She loses regular contact with her family. Her family loses her presence.

When couples separate, they are both still alive, but the relationship they hoped for, and the relationship they actually had, is lost. They must now negotiate life without the other. If there are children in the family, their way of life is also lost. They now have parents in separate houses, and often they have to go back and forth. Their sense of their family as one unit changes. There is a great deal of loss and a great deal of adaptation involved.

Ambiguous loss also occurs when a child has a new sibling. She may lose her place as an only child or her position as the youngest in the family. She loses some of her time with her parents, busy as they are with the new baby. They are still there—but their attention has refocused and usually the child feels this loss quite acutely.

Having a new sibling is what we would all consider a normal part of childhood—but it also contains a loss which deserves recognition. It is hard for children to share these feelings with their parents. The feelings that result from this experience, while not always discussed, can last a lifetime. I remember once asking my uncle, who was then in his eighties, what the worst thing was that had ever happened to him in his life. And he said, "It was when my younger sister was born." This had happened over eighty years ago and yet he still felt it was the worst thing that had ever happened to him!

Ambiguous loss also happens when a child waits for the birth of a sibling, and that baby dies before birth or at birth. There was never a baby to meet or to play with, so some people might say that there was no loss.

But there was.

The baby who was expected and planned for does not arrive. The child loses all the new possibilities and experiences that would have come with this new brother or sister. And the child may also lose her mother for a period while the mother grieves the lost baby.

In an essay in the *New York Times*, Teresa Pham-Carsillo describes what it was like after her mother had several miscarriages: "I always carried the awareness of the dead babies my mother mourned. I felt the responsibility of making up for their loss, of being five daughters in one body."[5]

Pham-Carsillo not only lost the siblings she might have had, but she also felt that she had to take care of her mother by making up for their loss.

Ambiguous loss even occurs when a child awaits a baby sibling, sure it will be a certain gender, and then it turns out that the baby is not that gender.

This sort of loss is much subtler than a loss due to death. But it is still painful, and it is still mourned by children and adults alike. These losses are not always acknowledged—and unacknowledged losses are harder for people to process.

When a loss goes unacknowledged, people may not even recognize that they have suffered a loss.

And even if they do realize their loss, many feel that they cannot talk about it openly.

As Pauline Boss says, "Ambiguous loss is always stressful and often tormenting."[6]

Children are more sensitive to changes in their lives than we often like to believe. When a child's sibling goes to college or joins the military or gets an apartment of their own, parents often fail to recognize that the child left at home may miss that sibling terribly. They may miss the way life was before. They may recognize that life will never be the same as it was when the whole family lived together. And for younger siblings in families of three or more children, this loss happens over and over as each older sibling leaves home. Eventually one child is left at home and life is indeed different from when there was the hustle and bustle of life with a full house.

Similarly, when a family moves to a different house or apartment—and/or to a different city or even a different country—the parents may be excited if it is a move to a better or a safer place, but the child may be sad because this means the loss of a familiarity, of the known. The child loses what they knew as home, they lose friends, they lose their school, teachers, and so many others. Children—and especially young children—love familiarity. A piece of furniture, for example, can be old and ratty, but it may still be their favorite place to curl up. Its smell, its feel, its place in a room can be comforting. And if given away, or left behind in a move, a child may miss it terribly for a while, just as they will miss other familiar places, objects, routines, and people.

In the decades following Boss's original research, she treated the families of Alzheimer's patients, families whose loved ones had died in natural disasters but whose bodies had never been recovered, and the families of those lost on 9/11. She said that for these families, their losses existed without any conclusion or resolution. She talked about the grief in these families as often being "frozen."

In frozen grief, there is sadness and longing but no moving forward in the grief process. There is no resolution or even partial resolution. Boss said, "Of all the losses experienced in personal relationships, ambiguous loss is the most devastating because it remains unclear, indeterminate . . . people hunger for certainty . . . the uncertainty makes ambiguous loss the most distressful of all losses, leading to symptoms that are often missed or misdiagnosed."[7]

For example, an eleven-year-old girl named Sophie came to see me when I worked at a community mental health clinic. While her father talked to a social worker, Sophie sat at a little child's table, even though she was tall with long legs. She wore leggings that bagged around her ankles and a rumpled dress. Her appearance left very little doubt that she was depressed.

Her father told me that he had no idea why his daughter was suddenly so sad. The thing that seemed to set off her sadness was that she had failed a French test. Normally an A student, she had broken down and cried for hours after she got her grade back.

When I went out to meet Sophie, I invited her to my office and tried to learn more about her. She had difficulty talking so I asked if she would like to make something with clay. She nodded her head "yes." She made a little house.

When I asked about it, she said it was her old house.

"Old house?" I asked.

"Yes," she said. She and her father and two brothers had recently moved from this old house to a different one.

Her father had not mentioned a move.

I asked her if she missed the old house, and again she nodded.

She then elaborated, saying that it was in that house that she had last seen her mother.

As it turned out, her mother had died by suicide in that house. And this had been three years ago.

However, this young girl's grief had been frozen.

Sophie's parents had been separated at the time of her mother's suicide, and her father had custody of the children. Her father had been very angry with her mother for several years because of her mother's drug use and neglect of the children. Her mother had come back to the house one day and argued with her father. She left the house, went to the garage, and killed herself.

Three years after her mother's suicide, the father and three children moved to an apartment, and Sophie continued to try her best to help her father with her younger brothers and to do well in school.

But she found that she had trouble concentrating on her schoolwork, something that had never been hard for her before. And when she failed her French test, she suddenly broke down. She wasn't sure why, and her father certainly did not know why.

But what we were able to put together was that losing the house triggered something for Sophie. She had last seen her mother at that house, and when she was little, her mother had lived in that house. The house linked her to her mother—and losing the house set all the grief she had not expressed over her mother's death in motion.

No one in her family understood that the loss of a house could have such meaning to her—and as such, no one understood her "sudden" sadness.

The loss of her house was an ambiguous loss for Sophie. It didn't seem like such a big deal. But it was. The house had symbolic resonances that had not been realized or acknowledged.

Another example of ambiguous loss is when a child is born with a chronic medical illness or disability or when they develop a chronic illness during childhood. This was described beautifully by Julie Kim in *The Atlantic*. She wrote about what she called "the loss of the future [she] imagined for [her] child."[8] In the article Kim described finding out that her unborn baby had a rare genetic condition that would limit her ability to develop the usual motor and intellectual milestones. Kim wrote eloquently about the loss she experienced. Her previous expectations for her daughter were irrevocably dashed.

When parents have a newborn with an illness or medical condition, the parents have not lost their baby. They have a new baby. But what they may have lost is the hoped-for baby. In this situation it is important for the parents to recognize their own lost expectations. As the baby grows, the parents are reminded of the fact that their expectations are not being met. They must mourn the loss of the "perfect" or even the "normal" baby/toddler/child they had envisioned. This is such a painful process—but one that must be acknowledged, felt, and spoken about.

In the case of Julie Kim, she still had a daughter, her son still had a sister. But the child each of them imagined coming into their home was not the child they actually had. And what about the inevitable alteration in the amount of time and attention the parents could give to their son? His life was undoubtedly changed by the presence of a sibling who has significant challenges. This is another sort of ambiguous loss.

What Kim did not mention in this essay is what this meant to the son she already had. Might he have looked forward to having a playmate, a sibling who would be able to do all the things he could do?

Ambiguous loss takes many forms. But whatever form it may take, it is best discussed openly; it is best acknowledged as a true loss, and it is best processed over time. It is helpful to children if parents and others can bring it up, talk about it, and share their own feelings about it.

PART 2

Helping the Grieving Child

Now that you've learned the different ways children of various ages experience and express their grief, and now that we have thought together about the different kinds of loss, you might be wondering how to penetrate the sadness of a child who is going through the mourning process and how to help them.

You certainly appreciate how hard this may be.

Fortunately, there are many different ways to help a child who has suffered the loss of a loved one.

And there is no single correct way.

Every child will experience loss in their own unique fashion. Each child will have their own individual way of understanding what has happened and their own particular way of responding.

We cannot pretend or imagine that there is a formula for helping children with their difficult feelings.

In this part of the book, I will talk about how to be with children who have experienced loss, how to know if a child needs help, and what you can do to help.

But first, I want to acknowledge that although we want to help children who are suffering, we must respect the fact that grief and mourning take time.

When we try to help a grieving child, we must do so knowing full well that they may not feel less bereaved, less lost, less sad, or less angry for quite a while.

We also understand that it does not help to try to distract them, to try to cheer them up, or to try to encourage them to hurry through their sadness and their upset—even though we might want them to move through their feelings quickly because it is so difficult for us to see them in pain.

What is necessary to help a grieving child is the courage to accompany them as they move through their sad and frightening feelings at their own rate.

What is also necessary is an attitude of patience, interest, and understanding.

In the chapters ahead I will talk about ways to approach children at each stage of development, I will provide concrete ideas for things you can do with the child, I will talk about how to recognize a child's need for professional help and what forms of professional help are available.

But before doing all of this, I would like to discuss something very difficult: how hard it is to help a grieving child when you yourself are bereaved.

CHAPTER 6

Understanding Your Own Grief

The cruel fact is that often those who are in the best position to help and support the bereaved child are also struggling with grief themselves.

If your spouse, your partner, your parent, your child, or your close friend has died, you will be in the middle of experiencing your own overwhelming feelings—and it will be hard, especially at first, to even consider the needs of your children.

You may feel that you *should* help your children and, in order to do so, you may be tempted to try to stay away from your own mourning.

However, your mourning process is important.

It is crucial for you to be able to feel what you feel for the period you need to feel it. You need to do this so that you will then be able to eventually move forward in your own life and in your ability to be a good parent.

There are just a few things you will need to do first:

- If you and your children have experienced the loss of a close loved one, tell your children about the loss yourself. It is best if you can do this directly and in person.
- It is also important to tell them how you feel. If you are feeling very sad or overwhelmed, tell them.
- If you feel like you cannot handle taking care of your children for the first few hours or days, ask someone to come in to help—and tell your children who it will be and what that person will be doing for them.

- Reassure your children that you will all be all right—even though you may not feel this way at the moment.

And after you have done all this, you will be freer to experience your own grief and to get the support you need.

Take time for yourself if you can.

And don't be afraid to reach out for help in your daily life. This is the best way that you can prepare yourself to also be able to care for and help your children.

Mourning is a labor-intensive process. Being sad, being in pain and feeling all the many feelings associated with loss leaves you with very little emotional energy to be of help to someone else, especially if that someone is a child.

And trying to push feelings of sadness and pain away is also very draining.

It may be hard to ask for help. It may feel impossible to let others know what you are going through. Your loss may be so profound that you may not even want to talk about it.

But it is of the utmost importance that you get all the help and support you can—both for your well-being and for your children's well-being. And you can seek that help in many different ways.

Here are just a few ideas to get the support you need after a loss:

- **Build time for yourself.** If you have family or friends who can be of help with childcare and who do not place additional stress on you or on your household, then you may need these people to step in for a few half or full days. Or you may need someone to take over more fully for a few weeks—or even for a few months while you grieve. If you have the financial resources, you may also choose to get any babysitters or nannies that you already employ to work more hours.
- **Reach out to a spiritual community.** If you have a spiritual community, even one that you were not particularly active in

previously, then allowing them to know what you are going through may be important for you—and possibly helpful for your family.

- **Set up a meal train or have a family member or friend do so for you.** Feeding a family can feel overwhelming when you are grieving. Friends, relatives, and church/synagogue/mosque communities are often willing to provide meals for a few weeks. Online platforms such as MealTrain.com or dedicated Facebook groups can help to organize this. In the longer term, if you have the resources, you can set up a meal service (HelloFresh, CookUnity, Dinnerly, Green Chef) to provide regular meals for your family—or you can ask a family member or friend to set this up for you.

- **Seek out professional help.** Sometimes it can be difficult to know how or where to begin the mourning process. A social worker, grief counselor, or therapist can provide emotional support for you, and they may also have ideas for helping you find caretaking and mealtime help in your area.

Finding a good therapist for yourself may be one of your first efforts at self-care. Having a place to express all of your feelings and begin to process them will help you to be more available to support your children in their grief and mourning process.

If you are not sure whether to get help, notice what you are feeling. Do you feel emotionally removed from your children? Are you having trouble with your daily caretaking activities? Do you feel anxious or depressed? And do you have enough social support? Reflecting on these questions can help you decide whether to try some therapy for yourself. And if you do want to seek out a therapist, start by asking others if they know of good therapists in your area or look on the *Psychology Today* website (https://www.psychologytoday.com/us/therapists) for local practitioners who specialize in working with people experiencing grief.

Try not to be afraid to ask for help; support is crucial during times of grief and mourning.

What Is Adult Mourning?

So, I have talked about what to do if you have experienced the loss of a loved one, but I have not talked about what mourning is like for adults.

If you have suffered the loss of a partner, parent, or child, or any close loved one, for that matter, your mourning may be intense and overwhelming—or it may be slow and steady.

It may come in powerful waves—or it may unfold slowly.

You may feel grief or sadness or numbness or anger or you may feel all of these in succession—or all of them at once.

Your feelings may overtake you immediately—or they may wait days or weeks or even months to show themselves.

Forget about the so-called stages of mourning.

Don't let anyone tell you how to feel or what you should be doing to mourn properly.

You will mourn at your own pace, in your own way.

Your mourning may involve a sense of shock at first. You may be asking yourself a million questions: How could this have happened? How could someone who was here yesterday be gone? How is this possible? And then: What do I do now? How can I go on?

You may feel that you are not up to the task of continuing your life. You may feel that you cannot go on.

This is normal. But usually, it is temporary.

After the initial shock usually comes a long period of experiencing so many strong feelings—sadness, anger, frustration, existential questioning. And also remembering.

You will be remembering the person you have lost and feeling all the feelings that these remembrances bring up.

This is called the work of mourning. It involves going through your memories one by one, sometimes when you least expect it: You will pass a familiar place and remember being there with your loved one. It will be a certain date and you will suddenly remember that that date had significance in your life with your loved one. You will eat a certain food and remember enjoying it with your loved one. You will watch your children and feel the absence of your loved one. You will plan an outing and forget that your loved one won't be there to go with you.

These memories and experiences can feel intensely painful. You may find yourself suddenly crying. You may be preoccupied with a multitude of memories, and feelings, with all the absences and the emptiness.

And again, this is normal.

And important. Reviewing your memories and letting yourself feel what you feel is what mourning is all about.

And mourning will take time and energy. It may take up to two years for you to begin to feel like yourself again.

Don't rush it. Allow it. Be gentle with yourself.

And remember, your mourning may *not* be filled with feeling and remembering. For a while, you may feel numb. You may feel less than you might have expected. If this is you, again, be patient with yourself. Your mourning may come on its own, or you may, at some point, decide to get some help to see what you are feeling.

Here are some ideas for things you can do to help yourself during this time:

- Seek out someone you can talk to—a friend, a sibling, a priest, rabbi, or imam.
- Share your grief—whatever form it is taking. Don't keep it all to yourself.
- Don't forget to eat. You may not feel like it, but you need to.

- Get out of the house. You may want to stay in. You may want to avoid the awkwardness of others, the looks of concern, the questions. But try to go out anyway.
- Have a stock answer ready when someone asks you how you are. If you don't feel like talking, just say, "It's hard" or "I'm managing."
- Let your children know how you are feeling. Don't be afraid to tell them, "I'm sad" or "I'm just so tired." They need to know.
- And when you are ready, check out the Resources section of this book. There are multitudes of wonderful books, podcasts, and other resources available that speak to loss and grief.

If you have feelings of sadness or hopelessness that persist, if you feel that you cannot go on, reach out. Call a friend or close relative. Let them help you get professional help.

You will feel better—but it may take some time.

And remember, over the coming years your children will need you. No matter how hopeless you feel, you still have a role in life, you are still important, you *can* feel better—and when you do, you can begin to help your children with *their* grief.

Below I provide some ideas about how to talk to them about your loss and theirs.

Communicating with Your Children

There have been many times in my practice when a parent who has been recently widowed or whose partner has experienced a catastrophic accident has come to me to ask how to help their children and how to move forward in their lives.

Like other therapists experienced in this area, I have been able to support these parents both in their own mourning and in talking to and helping their children.

Let me share some of the advice I've shared with my patients:

- Let your children in on what you are thinking and feeling. It is fine for them to see you in mourning.
- It is important for you to talk to them about feeling sad, or frustrated or angry or alone.
- It is fine to tell them about your memories of your lost loved one and what they make you feel.

If you do not talk to your children about what you are going through, they will develop their own theories about why you are sad and preoccupied.

Let me describe two people who came to me for help with their children after a major loss.

Simon was a young man who came to see me two weeks after his wife had been found in a coma. She had overdosed, and although she survived, she sustained significant brain damage.

She was now in a rehabilitation hospital. Simon's five-year-old son Charlie had not seen his mother since the overdose, and he had noticed that his father was sad and irritable all the time. The day after the overdose, Charlie asked his dad if he was mad at him,

This young father did not know what to tell his son about his mother—so he had not told him anything yet. He had a two-year-old to take care of as well, and it was all he could do to care for both of them while keeping up with his wife's medical condition over the phone.

Charlie did not know that his mother was in the hospital or that his father was very upset about this. So of course he filled in the gaps with the most logical explanation he could think of for why Daddy was sad and irritable—it was because he was angry with *him*.

I worked with Simon to be more open with his son about what had happened and about his own feelings. When we met, it was already two weeks after his wife's overdose, but we were able to talk together about how to begin to share more with Charlie in a way that he could understand and that would not be overwhelming to him.

So far, Simon had told him that Mommy was at work and would not be able to come back for a while.

I helped him to explain instead that Mommy was very sick and needed time to get better—and then to explain that Mommy was in a hospital and what a hospital is.

This young father was also not sure how to handle his two-year-old. He had not thought to talk with this child at all, feeling she would not understand. We talked about his toddler daughter's powerful missing-mommy feelings. We talked about how fussy she'd been recently and how she had resisted naps and bedtimes. I discussed with Simon how important it was to talk with both of his children, including his toddler, and to explain to both of them how he understood they were sad and missed their mommy.

I was also able to help Simon by asking him to talk about his own feelings. He told me that he was desperately sad. He missed his wife. But he was also angry. He had begged her to get help for her drug use, she had resisted, promising that she was no longer using . . . and then this had happened.

He was able to rage and cry with me for several sessions—and then he started to be able to focus more on his children's experience. We thought together about what each of his children might be feeling, and we spoke about how to address their sad feelings and their worries about where Mommy was and what had happened to her.

We discussed the importance of having both children see their mother on a regular basis, but how Simon would have to prepare them that Mommy would be different. He started by taking photos of his wife in her bed and in her wheelchair at the rehab hospital. He showed these to the children and named the different things in the pictures and why she needed them. He also explained why Mommy looked different.

After two days of doing this several times each day, he asked the children if they would like to go see Mommy—and they both indicated that they would.

When he took them to see their mother, they found her sitting in her wheelchair. Charlie ran to her and tried to give her a kiss while the two-year-old clung to Charlie and turned her head away from her mother.

After several minutes, Charlie asked for a ride in the wheelchair and climbed into his mother's lap. And then the two-year-old reached out toward her mother, seeming to want to be put on her lap as well. While their mother said little during this time, she allowed both children to sit on her lap while Simon pushed them around the rehab hospital for about fifteen minutes—and then they all went and got a cup of ice cream from the nurse's station.

This first visit was only around twenty-five minutes, but it was enough for the two children and for their mother, who was exhausted by the end.

While we only met six times, Simon felt helped by the chance to process some of his own feelings and by the opportunity to learn more about how children of five and two might experience the abrupt loss of their mother. Together we figured out how Simon could begin to talk with Charlie about his feelings and about his mother's condition and how Simon could also help his less verbal two-year-old.

I mentioned another widower who came to see me in chapter three when I wrote about blending families. His name was Matt, and he was a middle-aged professional man who came to my office several months after his wife had died. It was clear that he was in mourning—but at this point, he had enough energy to look into how to help his two children, ages eleven and fourteen.

What I initially thought would be several months of working together turned into several years.

Matt's children experienced tremendous sadness when their mother was ill and then when she died, and they continued to experience grief in all its forms for months and years. They missed their mother, they felt angry that she had to get sick and angry that the doctors could not cure her, they felt anxiety about what would happen if their father also died, and they each expressed these feelings in their own ways.

On many occasions in the years after their mother died, Matt's children had various reactions to what Matt considered common everyday events, and this confused Matt.

For example, as Matt wanted to make changes in their house, his children often wanted things to stay just as they had been when Mommy was there. He needed to replace some carpeting that was stained, but they objected. It seemed so clear to him that the carpeting needed to go, but his children saw it differently. He wasn't sure to whether to go through with the change or whether to give in to their desire to keep things the same.

In the end, he left the carpet as it was for the time being, realizing that he could replace it after a few months—or longer if necessary. He realized that the loss of his wife and his children's mother was still so fresh for all of them that it was not time to make any changes. He did not want to put his children through any more suffering than he had to.

As Matt progressed through his own mourning process, he found that his children had needs that were different from his. He struggled to give time and energy to himself while also caring for them. He came to talk with me every week to try to understand what each of his children might be experiencing, but he often left very little time in the sessions for his own feelings. We had to talk about it each time this happened so that he could begin to think about how to give himself some space for his own needs.

Matt endeavored to create ways of remembering his beloved wife, but his children sometimes did not want to participate or did not agree with the ways he was choosing to honor her. He wanted to visit the cemetery on a regular basis—and they did not. He wanted to set up a charity in her name—and his children had very little interest in hearing about it or in participating in any of the ceremonies associated with it.

We discussed these issues, and he was able to make room for both points of view. He was able to be patient with his children—allowing them to not participate—while also allowing himself to go forward with what he wanted to do.

And then, several years after his wife's death, Matt began to date. He kept his activities private for quite a while, but then he met someone and became involved in a committed relationship—and he let his children know about what was happening.

Each of his children had a great deal of trouble with this.

His daughter worried that Matt would no longer love her. And this worry did not go away with his reassurances. She continued to ask him, over and over again, if he loved her.

And his son felt that Matt was being disloyal. The son was angry and refused to talk with Matt's new partner.

With each of these situations there was a lot for us to talk about in our sessions. We needed to talk about how to understand each of the children's reactions, how to deal sensitively with their feelings, how to honor Matt's own process of moving forward in his life, and how to be sensitive to the feelings of his partner.

The work Matt and I did together was complex. Over the years, his children's needs changed, as did his own. He needed to continue to be sensitive to his children's feelings while also establishing some limits with them. As time went by, he needed to allow more space for the exploration of his own grief and later, for developing an openness to moving forward in his own life.

As was the case for these two grieving men, handling your own grief and that of your children is a process. It occurs over weeks and months and years. You learn as you go, and you do the best you can. And if you need help, you reach out to those who can provide some of what you need.

Grief Modeling

Besides trying to understand what you are feeling and what your children are feeling, as the parent or close relative of grieving children, besides talking to them and besides getting support for yourself and for them, you are also a role model. Your children will be watching to see how you deal with your own sad feelings.

You may be afraid to cry in front of them. You may think it is better not to display your own feelings or even to talk about them.

Crying or talking about your feelings in front of children who are also grieving is not necessarily the wrong thing to do. It is natural that you will have your own strong feelings, and the way you deal with these will show your children one way that they might be able to deal with their own feelings.

If you are able to cry in front of your children without feeling out of control—that is, if you are able to cry while you are in the same room with your children without showing them the most overwhelming or dramatic of your feelings, which may scare them—you may be surprised to see that your children will accept this. They may come to comfort you, and they may also be willing to cry in front of you.

Children need to feel that expressing feelings through tears or words is an acceptable thing to do in your family. They may like to feel that they can be a comforter or helper as well as someone who is comforted and helped.

In my own family, there was very little expression of feelings. After my father died, I did not see my mother or my sisters cry even once. Did the fact that they did not cry have anything to do with my own inability to cry very much about my father's death?

I suspect it did.

Children need role models for the expression of grief. As a parent or close relative, you are one of the people the child will be closely observing. You will be one of the people the child will look to for how to grieve and how to express grief.

To summarize, here are some key points:

- Talk to your children about how you feel about your loss. Keep doing this from time to time as the weeks and months and years go by.
- Let your children see you cry if you happen to feel like crying while they are in the room.
- Let yourself feel your most dramatic feelings when your children are not home or not in the room, if possible.
- Don't be afraid to ask for help from loved ones or seek professional help.

CHAPTER 7

How to Help a Grieving Child

In this chapter, I will talk about the specifics of how to help children of various ages who have suffered loss.

But first, remember—I am not trying to suggest that there is a single right way to help a grieving child at any stage.

As I mentioned earlier, each child will experience loss in their own unique way. And each person trying to help a grieving child will have their own particular approach. Each person will have something special they can offer.

And as I also mentioned previously, we cannot pretend or imagine that there is a formula for helping children with their difficult feelings.

And it's hard even to try. We can feel awkward, we can fear saying the wrong thing, we can freeze and feel inadequate. We can also be tempted to turn away from a child's pain because of how difficult it is for us to understand what the child is feeling—or because it evokes memories for us of our own losses.

However, in this section I will offer helpful ideas, tools, and suggestions.

Your approach and your attitude are important.

No matter the age of the child, the most important tool you need to begin to help is the desire to understand what the child is feeling.

You simply cannot expect yourself to know what feelings a grieving child is having, how intense these feelings are, or what kind of help will be best.

As you know from reading part 1, the grieving child will be experiencing any combination of feelings. And their feelings may be quite different from those you would expect them to be having. They may be confused and find it difficult to understand what has happened. They may be angry at having been left. They may feel all alone and abandoned by the person who has died and/or by the other family members who are also grieving. They may be frightened by what they are experiencing inside of themselves, by the behavior of the other grieving people in their lives, or by the actual events surrounding their loss. They may try to hide all their feelings to look OK to others. They may be shut down emotionally and reluctant to even admit to feelings.

But in your effort to help, you can communicate your wish to understand what the child is experiencing, whatever that may be.

You can communicate your wish to understand through your attitude of interest, your open-mindedness toward what the child's experience might be, and through a sensitive and gentle attempt to explore their feelings with them. This in and of itself is extremely helpful.

Children usually like to feel that someone is interested in them and in what their experience is.

Here are some key steps to take to work toward understanding what your child is going through and establishing a level of trust so that they are able to accept your support.

Step 1: Tell the child you want to know what they're feeling.

For children over the age of three, you will want to convey that you are available to them and that you are interested. Depending on what your relationship is with the child, there will be a variety of ways to do this. As a parent or close relative, you can tell the child directly that you want to hear all about what they are feeling.

Be sure to avoid telling them what they *should* feel and what they should *not* feel. In other words, try not to say things like "We all feel sad right now" or "Don't worry about that."

For younger children such as toddlers or for children who do not respond well to direct communication, you can simply sit down with them to play. Do this as often as you have time to, and see what emerges in the play. Are there themes of loss or illness in what they are playing? Do they play out scenes where one character goes to the doctor or where one character looks for another and cannot find them? Is one of the characters sad? Or angry? If so, you can comment gently on this, "Oh! I see the elephant is very sad/angry that he cannot find his friend." You do not have to take it any further than this to start with. Just notice the feelings that come up in the play and name them.

For an older child, whether you are a parent or a relative or a close friend of the family, you can offer to play a game with the child on as many occasions as you are able, and see what conversation comes up during the game.

You can also just go through your usual activities with the child—meals, outings, driving in the car—and be alert to the child's mood, to what she talks about—and comment, again gently, about what she seems to be feeling.

This may not sound like much, but it is the beginning of letting the child know that feelings can be named and talked about and that you are willing and available to do so with her.

Step 2: Get personal about your own experiences.

Again, for children over the age of about three, when the child is interested and listening, you can bring up some of your own experiences with loss and how you feel or felt.

Children often like to discover that they are not alone in what they are experiencing. If you were close to the person the child has lost, you can bring up some of your own feelings about their death. If you were not close to them, you can bring up an example of someone that you lost in your life, especially if this happened when you were around the same age as the child. You will see whether the child is curious to find out how you felt and how you handled your loss.

But take your cues from the child. If she does not respond with interest, drop the subject. If she starts to ask you questions, bingo! You know you have succeeded in helping her to feel less alone.

Answer her questions, but keep in mind that your goal is to share only as much as may be helpful to her. For example, you might say, "I was around your age when my mother died," and then wait to see how she responds.

If the child asks, "What did you do?" tell her the truth. You can say, "Well, I didn't know what to do" or "I felt very sad for a long time." Do not try to sugarcoat your experience. Children need to know that others have suffered pain like their own and that they have survived it.

Step 3: Remember to listen more than you talk.

Giving long speeches to children is seldom helpful. Try to listen to what the child has to say no matter what she is talking about. This will convey your interest—and if she does not bring up her feelings about her loss right away, it is more likely that she will do so eventually if she knows you are listening.

Try to tolerate hearing about sad feelings or sad experiences. Resist the urge to "fix" the situation. Do not try to come up with suggestions to make things better. The sadness that a child feels after a loss is not something that can be fixed.

Here is a summary of ways to begin to establish trust with a grieving child and to communicate your interest in their feelings and experience:

- **Be available.** Spend time with the child, listen to the child, talk about your own feelings when you have experienced loss.

- **Be vulnerable.** Be open to sharing your experiences with your child so that they don't feel so alone.
- **Listen more, talk less.** Listen to what the child has to say and the questions the child has. Talk about your own feelings only if you think the child would like to hear from you or if you think they need help figuring out how to feel and how to mourn.

Helping Children at Each Age

We all know that the needs of children vary depending on their age and stage of development, and this is true for children who have experienced a loss as well.

In part 1, I went through how loss affects children at each age and stage of development. Here I will describe some of the things that can be done at each age that may be helpful if a parent or other close relative has died.

But for children of every age, from infancy through late adolescence, there are certain things which will apply universally. Let me start with these.

- **Be honest.** After infancy, all children need to be told about the death of a close family member promptly, honestly, and face to face. If a parent is not available to tell them, have someone they are familiar with tell them the news. Tell them in terms they can understand. And if there is something that is not yet known, just tell them that.

    At times people feel it is better not to tell children certain things. They believe that they are "protecting" the child. There are several problems with this idea. First, children are often very perceptive, and they will know when we are hiding something or telling less than the whole story. Second, often children already know the answers to their questions, they are just making sure that they are right. Third, if we do not tell the children the whole story, they are likely to hear the parts we have not told them elsewhere and their trust in us will be undermined.

So if a child asks how Daddy died, it is important to answer the question in a way that is appropriate to their age and stage of development but still truthful. For example, if a parent died of an illness, at times the surviving parent is afraid to mention the details of what happened. They worry that these details may scare the child, they may make the child worry about their own health or the health of others, or they may cause them to lose faith in doctors and hospitals.

However, there is often a way to answer. For a younger child, you can say, "Daddy was very, very sick and the doctors tried very hard to help him, but sometimes even doctors are not able to help enough."

For an older child, you can name the illness and tell them a little bit about it. If they are interested, you can tell them more about it and how the doctors tried to treat the illness.

Be aware of what the child may have already overheard and bring this up. For example, you might say, "I know you've heard us talk about Daddy's heart attack—well, what happened was that Daddy's heart suddenly stopped working in the right way," etc.

Or if the person died in an accident, you can simplify the details while still retaining the truth.

If the person died of old age, you can tell the child about this and reassure them, if this was the case, that at the end of life people are often very, very tired and unable to do many of the things they used to do, that their bodies are worn out, and that they are ready to die.

And if the person died by suicide? This is a difficult subject for anyone, let alone a child. When one parent has died by suicide, the surviving parent often struggles with whether to tell the children. They worry that the child will feel responsible for the parent's death, or that the child will think that suicide is a viable option for how to handle difficult feelings. For more on this subject, you can refer back to chapter 4.

Depending on what the child has witnessed or overheard about how their loved one died, you will tailor your answers to their questions according to their level of curiosity and the degree to which they can understand the complexities.

While it is important not to frighten the child, it is, again, important to be truthful. This way, the child will know that you can be trusted.[1]

- **No matter the age of the infant, child or teen, try to stick to familiar routines after the loss.** Children of all ages are comforted by routine. While it is natural that the first few days after a loss will be chaotic, try to return to the normal order of things to the extent possible as soon as you can. Regular mealtimes, homework times, and bedtimes can provide a sense of security for children.

- **If childcare is needed, have familiar caregivers come in.** Try to keep the familiar rhythms and practices going. If less familiar people volunteer to come help out, try to get one or two to take most of the time needed, if possible. Having multiple caretakers can feel chaotic and upsetting for some children.

- **If there is trouble with sleep, keep to the normal bedtime, but be flexible with the sleeping arrangements for a little while.** Infants and toddlers may need more holding before naptime and bedtime. Children may need someone to sit with them while they go to sleep. They may even need the option of bringing some pillows or a sleeping bag into a sibling's room or the parent's room for a while.

- **Never force a child to talk about the person who has died.** But feel free to talk about that person yourself, in front of the child. And, as discussed in chapter 6, feel free to express your feelings in words to the child.
- **Answer all the child's questions, no matter how difficult.** Whether you are the grieving child's parent, close relative, teacher, or friend, if the child asks you a question about her loss, answer it.
- **Expect the child to bounce in and out of their grief.**[2] Don't expect the toddler, child, or teenager to be sad all the time. Children are often sad for a few minutes when they are thinking of the loved one they lost and then they may go back to their usual activities.[3]
- **Bring in others to help.** The child needs all the help he or she can get at this time. If she gives you permission, tell her teacher about the loss and ask the teacher to be sensitive to the feelings your child may be having, which may affect her performance and/or behavior in school. Bring in others who love the child—aunts, uncles, grandparents, cousins, family friends—to provide additional support. Bring in a therapist to help the family and/or the child if necessary.
- **Respect the child's feelings.** If she prefers to spend some time alone, allow it. If she prefers to not talk about the loss for a few weeks, allow it.
- **Seek a professional evaluation from a grief specialist, psychologist, or social worker.** If your child will not talk about the loss or prefers to spend time alone for more than a period of several weeks to a few months, seek professional help.

Now let's look at how you can more specifically help a child depending on their age.

The Newborn (Zero to Four Months)

For the youngest infants, the only loss that will directly impact the baby is the loss of a parent, particularly the primary caretaker. So what can you do for a young infant who has experienced the loss of a parent and/or for the family when the parent of a young infant dies?

It may be hard to believe, but as you read in part 1, even young infants can be affected by the loss of a parent. They can perceive changes in their caretaking routines, and they are aware of the deep feelings in their caretaker. If that caretaker is sad and grieving, they will likely be affected by this.

Or if they are suddenly taken care of by someone new, they will feel the difference in the way they are held, the way they are fed, and the way they are soothed. These new ways may feel less comforting to them than the old, familiar ways.

They may react by being fussy or out of sorts, by eating less or more, by sleeping less or more, by digestive upset, and by other signs of bodily dysregulation.

What is most helpful, unfortunately, is also most difficult following the loss of a parent or caretaker—and that is to try to maintain stability for a young infant.

As I said above, it is best if the same few caretakers care for them. If the infant needs to be looked after by someone other than their familiar caretaker, it is best if someone else familiar can take over and be the main caregiver. But, unfortunately, in the panic following a loss, it is often a matter of finding someone—anyone—to care for the baby.

The issue here is that infants thrive on routine and stability, and when this is in very short supply, they may suffer.

If you are the parent of an infant and you have lost your partner, you will be in survival mode. You will just be doing your best to get through each day. All you can do is provide as much love and care and routine for your infant as you possibly can—and then try to bring in others who can love and care for your baby on as regular a schedule as you can manage.

You may feel overwhelmed. And this is totally understandable. In addition to caring for your baby you will need to take care of yourself and find places where you can express and experience all of your feelings safely and in comfort. As I mentioned earlier, going through your own grief process will be the best thing you can do for yourself—and in the long run, it will also be the best for your baby. Talking with friends or family, engaging in psychotherapy, or even joining an online community maybe helpful (see Resources, page 255).

If you are a relative or friend of a family in which there has been the loss of a parent or primary caregiver of a young infant, it is crucial to do your best to ensure that the surviving parent or caregiver receives as much love and support as possible.

When a parent dies or leaves the family, the remaining parent will be placed under a great deal of strain. In addition to their own inevitable grief process, they will also experience a dramatic increase in the number of responsibilities they must take care of. Under these circumstances, one of the best things you can do for the baby or children in the family is to support their remaining parent. If this parent becomes depressed or overstressed, the effects on the children may be severe—because in this case, they have effectively lost both parents.

See if you can set up a meal train. Pitch in or find someone to help with laundry, cleaning, grocery shopping, and babysitting. You can also offer emotional support instead of or in addition to any of these things.

It is often the case that the parent of a young infant who has been bereaved does not even know what they need.

Instead of asking them to tell you when you are needed, just offer to help in a specific way, such as bringing meals weekly or taking over a household task—and stick to it beyond the first few weeks after the death. The needs of the bereaved parent will continue for weeks or months after their loss.

In brief, here are the most important things you can do for a young infant who has suffered a loss:

- If you are not the parent, provide extra support for the parent(s) at this time.
- If you are the parent, try to keep caretaking routines as consistent as possible. Provide as much extra cuddling and soothing to your infant as possible. You may find that this is soothing for you as well.
- Bring in the help you need but make sure to try to keep the number of caretakers as small as you can. Help them to know what routines the baby is used to. Encourage them to provide extra cuddling, holding, and soothing.

Older Infants (Four to Eight Months)

If an infant of four to eight months of age loses their primary caretaker, the things you can do to help are much like the things suggested for the younger infant.

But something to consider is that when I talk about a four-to-eight-month-old losing their primary caregiver, I am not talking only about the loss of a parent. The loss of a nanny or a babysitter who came every day—or even several days a week—is also a *big* loss for an infant of this age. While such a loss may not feel like a big deal to other family members, to the infant of this age the nanny or babysitter was a very important person. The four-to-eight-month-old will be affected by the absence of their familiar person, they will miss her, and things will feel very different for quite a while without her.

It is important to recognize the significance of the loss of a nanny or babysitter for the baby—and it can be helpful to talk about and acknowledge this with the baby—even if it feels strange to do this with a four-to-eight-month-old.

You can begin to name the baby's feelings in a very simple way. If a baby of this age calls out for a nanny who has left, the caretaker who is present can name that feeling, saying for example, "Oh, you want Catherine. Catherine isn't here. You miss her so much. You feel sad." The baby may cry when this is said, but that does not mean that this is the wrong thing to say. It is important to allow the baby to feel sad, to learn the meaning of the word "sad," and to connect that word to what she feels. This is far better than trying to distract the baby from thinking about the loved one who is gone.

For example, Teddy had a wonderful babysitter named Tracy from the time he was three months old until he was just under a year. Tracy loved Teddy. She was a very creative person who played in all sorts of clever ways with him, who helped him learn to sit up and crawl, who made up games, and laughed and had a lot of fun with him every day. She was also good at soothing him and at getting him to take his naps.

But as he approached nine months old, Teddy just became too heavy for Tracy to lift and carry. Tracy was an older woman who had had terrible back pain for a number of years. She was very sad to leave the family, and they were very sad to lose her. Of course Teddy did not understand that Tracy would not be caring for him every day any-more. And after she left for the last time, a new babysitter, Christa, took Tracy's place. Teddy accepted Christa after a few days of shyness and fussiness—but he had had a real relationship with Tracy and her absence was undoubtedly disturbing to him. For everyone's sake, Tracy and Teddy's family kept up contact. Teddy's mother and father frequently talked about Tracy to Teddy, and they made the trip to her house to see her once every few months. Teddy always recognized Tracy and was excited to see her. In fact, once he got to be around two and a half, he was the one to start to ask for visits with her.

In this case, Teddy's loss was not complete. His family was able to support a continued connection with his wonderful babysitter and this was helpful to Teddy.

But in the case of a more total loss—including a death—it is also extremely important for the parent to remember the person who has died with the baby, "Oh, you're thinking of Grandma. You're sad you can't see her. I'm sad too." And throughout that baby's development, the lost loved one can be remembered and talked about, photos can be looked at, and stories can be told.

Most importantly, throughout the child's development, the parents can provide the message that it is all right to be sad, that we can miss people and remember people and tolerate these difficult feelings.

For a four-to-eight-month-old, other losses will also be noticed— for example, if an older sibling goes to sleep-away camp—the parent can help the infant to understand what has happened through repetition. "Your sister is away at camp! You miss her! So do I." If the infant calls her name or indicates that he wants to see his sister, the parent can also put these feelings into words, "Oh, you're thinking about your sister!" And the parent can provide reassurance, "She's coming back! You'll see her soon!"

It is much better to acknowledge a loss, even if it happens early in a baby or child's life, than to pretend it did not happen or that it did not affect the baby or the child in any way.

After a loss, it is also important, as I stated at the beginning, to keep routines at home as consistent as possible. This provides the infant of this age a sense of continuity and safety. It is also important to give the infant who has experienced a loss as much extra love and support as can be managed.

In brief, here are some things you can do for the baby who has suffered a loss:

- If you are not the parent, provide the parents with extra support during this time.
- If you are the parent, do your best to provide the baby with patient, loving caretaking, whether from you or from the person doing the caretaking.

- Keep the caretaking routines as consistent as possible.
- Provide extra cuddling, soothing, and holding during this time.
- Put the baby's feelings into words.

Older Infants (Eight Months to One Year)

From the age of approximately eight months to a year old, babies experience more feelings associated with loss. They are more aware of being a separate person at this age, different from their parent or caregiver. They are more independent, now able to scoot or crawl or walk, and they are sensitive to being apart from the people they depend on.

If a parent or caregiver who previously cared for them and loved them is gone, they will long for the lost loved one, they will protest the loss through angry behavior or crying, and after a week or two, they may show signs of despair such as listlessness, sleepiness, or a lack of desire to play or eat. If an adequate substitute caretaker is not provided, they may also start to detach themselves both from their own feelings and from their relationships with others. This represents a dangerous deterioration in functioning and requires immediate help.

In order to prevent this detachment and deterioration, the best thing you can do for the child of this age, as with the younger infant, is to make sure they have good substitute caretaking. If a parent has died, try to find one or two people who can care for the one-year-old on a regular basis and provide extra love and nurturing. If you are the caretaker, provide as much love and support as possible. Imitate the lost parent's caretaking as closely as possible. Talk to the child about their feelings. If there are signs that the child is missing the lost loved one—or searching for them—talk to them about what they are doing and what they are feeling.

And as with the younger baby, keep routines as consistent as possible. This provides the infant of this age a sense of continuity and safety.

In brief, here are several things you can do to help the child of eight months to one year who has suffered a loss:

- If you are not the parent, support the parents in any way possible, both emotionally and by providing help in the way of meal preparation, babysitting, and so on.
- If you are the parent or a close loved one, put the baby's feelings into words for her when she seems to be reacting to the loss with sadness, frustration, or fussiness.
- If it is the parent or beloved caretaker who has left or died, encourage all of those who care for the baby to provide extra cuddling and soothing as well as patient, loving care.

Older Infants to Toddlers (One to Three Years)

If you are the parent of a toddler who has suffered a loss, you will notice that they may be fussy or sad at times, they may yearn to see their lost loved one, they may look for them, they may run around the house searching for them, they may go to familiar places where they last saw their loved one, and/or they may ask for them. They are much more aware of and sensitive to separations than an infant—and they are better able to express their distress.

Yearning and searching for a lost loved one is all part of normal grieving for a toddler. This is their way of remembering and trying to reclaim their lost loved one.

And the best thing you can do is to accompany them emotionally as they go through these feelings. "Maybe you're thinking of Grandma—this is the time she came over every day—you're looking for her! You miss her! But she can't come anymore. It's so sad." Then give a big hug.

This will not make the fussiness or the sadness or the yearning and the searching go away necessarily, but it will validate your toddler's feelings and help her to name and understand them herself.

If you are not the parent, but a toddler in your life has lost a loved one, particularly a parent, a sibling, or a close grandparent, the very best thing you can do, as mentioned previously, is to support the grieving parent(s). Providing the parent(s) with additional love and help will enable them to be more available for their toddler.

Depending on your relationship with the family and with the toddler herself, you can also provide extra love and attention to the child. If you are close to the family, and if you have the time to devote to the child, offer to babysit or to spend a half day or more per week with the child. This will give the parent(s) a chance to do something for themselves, and it will provide an additional relationship for the child to draw on in her life. Reading books, doing little projects, playing and being open to the child's concerns about life and death can be very helpful.

Purchasing a couple of very elementary books about death and giving them to the family may also be helpful (see the Resources section of this book for ideas).

Even small children can be aware of a grieving parent's fragility. If a child's parent has lost their partner or their own parent or if they have lost a child, they will be grieving and this will affect the one-to-three-year-old. The toddler will notice that their parent is not the same. They will pick up on sad or anxious feelings, and they may feel that it is their job to comfort their parent or to distract them from their sadness and anxiety. Of course, this is not optimal for the toddler, and it may be beneficial at this point for them to start at preschool or to spend time with a loving adult who is not mourning to get some extra love and to explore their feelings and worries.

But perhaps most important for the child of this age are frequent gentle explanations. They can be helped to understand the feelings of their grieving family members, and they can also be helped to understand why the loved one who has died is no longer available to them. They will need help understanding death, and simple explanations will be important. They can be told that the loved one who has died *cannot* come back. The toddler has difficulty understanding the idea of permanence, and she has trouble understanding that it was not her fault that her loved one went away. She needs frequent reminders that it was not her fault *and* that Mommy/Daddy/Grandpa would come back if they could because they would want to be with her, but they cannot because they have died.

Mourning starts with the acceptance that the loved one has died and is never coming back, and the toddler needs abundant help keeping this in mind.

Also, as development progresses, the child's inner resources increase; the young child can experience loss in an increasingly sophisticated way. One of the primary differences in the response to loss in early childhood versus later childhood, adolescence, and adulthood is the ability to independently reorganize. Toddlers and young children do not have this ability, and as a result, they need a great deal of help from the adults around them to do this. When they are fussy, when they are sad, when they are remembering the person they have lost, they need the adults around them to soothe them and to talk with them until they are able to calm down and regain a sense of well-being.

In brief, here are the things you can do to help the young toddler who has suffered a loss:

- If you are not the parent, provide extra support for her parent(s) during the weeks and months following the loss.
- Put the toddler's feelings into words for her.
- Answer all her questions simply and honestly.
- Explain death as often as you need to.
- Purchase a few elementary books on death and read them to her now and then.
- Try to be patient with repeated questions.
- Soothe the toddler when she is sad until she is able to calm down again.
- Tell her teachers what has happened and ask them to be sure to provide extra support to her.

Three to Four Years Old

The best things that can be done for a three-to-four-year-old who has lost a loved one are to give her extra love and support and to help her to understand what has happened.

The three-to-four-year-old is generally quite social and well connected to those she loves. She will miss loved ones who must leave or who die, quite intensely, but she will also understand much better than the younger toddler what death means when it is explained to her. She will remember seeing dead bugs and dead animals. She will more readily accept explanations about what happened to the person who has gone and why they had to die or leave her.

But she will still be prone to forgetting the real story, and she will tend to develop her own fantasies about what has happened. She will need to be reminded frequently of the truth of the matter. And she will need soothing and help to calm herself when she is sad.

It will help the three-to-four-year-old who attends daycare or school if her teachers are informed about what has happened and if they are on board with providing extra support during the weeks and months following the loss.

In brief, here are several ways to help the three-to-four-year-old:

- **Explain what has happened concretely.** For example, you can say, "It is very sad but today Grandma died. Now she cannot come over anymore. She cannot eat or sleep or breathe anymore. This is what happens when someone dies."
- **Use examples of others who have died to remind the child what death is.** You can talk about other people she has known who have died or even animals and bugs she may have seen that have died.[4] Emphasize that people who have died cannot come back again.
- **Give examples of feelings she may feel in the next few days.**[5] You can say, "Over the next few days you might feel very sad or lonely or even angry."

- **Answer all her questions—no matter how often she asks them.** Children of this age need to hear the same stories over and over to absorb them. This helps the child of this age to think realistically rather than relying on her own fantasies and imagination.

- **Tell her a little about how you feel or have felt at other times when someone has died.** Talk about people you have lost and how you felt.

- **Prepare the child for the grief rituals that will be taking place.**[6] Assign someone to sit with the child if she attends the funeral. This person should be someone with whom the child has a prior relationship and who can explain what is going on and take her outside if she needs to take a break or to leave during the service.[7]

- **Understand that after a loss, separations from the parent(s) of more than a day will be very difficult for several months following the loss.**[8] The child of this age will need to be prepared several days in advance if a parent is going away, and they will need reassurance that the parent is coming back. Sometimes making a calendar showing the days the parent will be away is helpful and allowing the child to cross off each day as it goes by can be a very concrete way for them to see that the time is coming when the parent will return. Having face time on the phone can also be helpful while the parent is away—and while the child may be sad or cry during or after the face time, this does not mean it is a bad idea to do it. Continual reassurance that the parent is still alive and will come back is necessary as the child of this age may be confused about the difference between a temporary departure and death.

- **Find ways to remember the loved one who has been lost and encourage the child to participate.** Perhaps you can light a special candle at holidays or make a special toast to them. If the child is willing, go to the cemetery to visit from time to time. Let the child leave flowers or place a stone on the grave. Or just tell stories at home about the loved one from time to time.[9]

It is important to remember that even a three-to-four-year-old may imagine that other people's sadness is their fault. They may think they have done something bad to cause the sadness they see a parent or grandparent feeling. It is important to make sure that they know the actual reason why the other people in their family are sad.

Children as young as three can also think it is their job to make people feel better. And they may be very worried when they see loved ones who are deep in their grief. While the development of this sort of empathy and desire to help is a very positive thing, it can go too far. It is important to make sure that there is someone available to care for and reassure the young child and to help other people in the family have access to support aside from the young children in the family.

Raymond was three when his father died quite suddenly. His mother was devastated and was unable to function for weeks after her husband's death. Raymond's grandmother came in to take care of them both—but she was unable to get Raymond to go to preschool. He cried and cried in the mornings and said he didn't want to go. For the first week she allowed him to stay home. Raymond's mother stayed in bed that week and what Raymond did for most of the day was to sit on his mother's bed while she slept and watched TV.

The following week, Raymond's grandmother again tried to take him to school. And again he cried and refused. He said he wanted to be with Mommy.

Raymond was very confused and frightened. Daddy had left and not come back, and he was very afraid of losing Mommy. He was also very frightened by how changed his mother was. She lay in bed all day and didn't do any of her usual activities.

In the third week after his father's death, Raymond's mother was able to get up and get dressed. She started to make breakfast for all of them, and when it was time to go to preschool, she got in the car with Raymond and her mother—and he agreed to go.

Raymond seemed happy and relieved to see his mother functioning again. While it is hard to know exactly what allowed him to go back to preschool, it is likely that once he could stop worrying about his mother, once she was able to resume some of her usual activities, he was able to resume his own usual routine, to go to preschool, and to separate from her.

Four to Five Years Old

The four-to-five-year-old child who has suffered the loss of a close loved one needs help to understand what has happened—and many of the suggestions already provided will apply. But at this age they are more aware of the world around them than the younger child, and they will easily pick up on anything they overhear or learn indirectly about the loss.

As a result, it is important for children starting at this age to be told clearly what has happened as soon as possible after it has happened. They will have innumerable questions, and these should be answered simply and factually.

But the four-to-five-year-old will need more help with feelings. They will readily express their own opinions, but around loss they may need some help putting their feelings into words.

Children of this age are curious, and they will often ask the same questions over and over. This is true when it comes to death and loss as well, and this can be difficult for the adults around them. But as *Helping Children Cope with Death*, a wonderful book from the Dougy Center, points out, children of this age learn by repetition.[10] Just as they watch the same movie again and again, they may want to repeatedly hear what happened to the person who died.

Children of this age, like the younger child, can also be convinced that the death itself was their fault or the sadness that others are demonstrating around the loss has something to do with what they have or have not done. Some basic explanation of why people are sad when someone dies can be helpful.

And, as with the younger child, when children of this age try to comfort their siblings or the adults in their family, this can be noticed and praised—but also limited. It is not the job of the young child of four or five to take care of other family members.

To help the four-to-five-year-old:

- Remind the child of the facts of what has happened and why.
- Make sure that any fantasies the child has about why the death occurred are corrected repeatedly.
- Make sure the adults in the family have adequate support so that they do not have to lean on their young child for comfort.

I learned about the importance of this last point in my conversation with Lucine, a young adult who had many losses in her early life. This is what she told me:

Around five, six, I became the main support in my family. A sibling was born and there were a couple of deaths on my mother's side so parenting was difficult for her. I had to be there for her. I became quite numb. . . . I was aware of sadness but I couldn't tap into it then . . . I didn't have the full concept, I couldn't really do anything with the feelings in me because I had to do so much. I went through my childhood and teen years just like, yeah, there's a lot of sadness but there wasn't a lot of understanding—it was distant . . . like it was across the road.

It is hard to imagine Lucine as a five-year-old having to be a support to her mother, but this is not so unusual. Sometimes a parent who has been bereaved has intense needs and very few people to go to. In such situations, a parent may invite her young child to sleep in bed with her thinking that this is for the child's comfort, when it may also be for the parent's comfort. Or a parent will ask a young child to play with her younger siblings for a great deal of the day in order to allow the parent some grieving room.

As a grieving parent, if you are in such a situation, try to be aware of the effect your requests of your child have on her. And try to find others to support you and your young children.

If you are a family member or friend of a family where a loss has occurred, try to be a support for the grieving parent so that they do not have to rely so much on their young child.

Friends and extended family can be of help by offering more love and attention to the parent as well as to the child.

It is also important to be aware that often children can feel sidelined by all the preparations for a funeral and all the attention paid to the adults in the family. But it is extremely important to remember that they are also deeply affected by what is going on, and needful of acknowledgement that they are having their own difficult experience.

Here are some ways friends and family can help:

- Offer to babysit for a few hours at a time.
- Bring over art supplies and do some drawing or other creative activity with the children in the family.
- Suggest to the child or children that they may want to make cards for the people in the family who are sad. Children of this age love to make things and they also love to give little gifts to people.
- If they seem open to it, talk to the child about times you have lost someone you loved.
- Talk about the feelings you have when you are grieving.

Six to Eleven Years Old

When a loved one dies, the child of this age understands what has happened. Usually they already have a good understanding of death. But they may have a lot of questions about what happened, how it happened, and why it happened.

At this age, children also often want to be of help. And it is better for them to have an active role in the grief process than to sit by passively.

They can be given jobs to do. They can be asked to make cards for others who are grieving. They can take on new jobs around the house—and they may be proud to do so.

Also, at this stage of development, learning is all-important—children are interested in how the world works and they are endlessly curious. They will use their intellect to understand why and how their loved one died, and they may put energy into trying to figure out how to prevent others from dying or leaving them.

It will be helpful to talk to the child of this age often about what has happened and what they are feeling.

When talking with a six-to-eleven-year-old who has suffered a loss:

- Make sure to ask the child what questions she has.
- Answer her questions honestly, to the extent that is appropriate at this stage of development. For example, if she asks why people have to die, you can answer the question concretely as you would for a younger child, saying that all living things die eventually, and this includes all of the natural world—plants, animals, sea creatures, and so on. You can explain, as you would for a younger child, that when a person dies, they stop breathing, they stop eating, sleeping, seeing, hearing, and being conscious. You can tell them that all bodily processes stop. But you can also answer on the more spiritual level, according to your own beliefs and those of the child's

family. When you do so, tell the child that these are your beliefs, and let the child know that she can also ask others what they believe and that she can develop her own beliefs.

- If the child wants to know about how their parent or close loved one died, tell them honestly. If they want to know details about the illness or accident, tell them in terms that are true but not overly lurid.
- Avoid trying to "look on the bright side" or telling the child "well, at least you still have your father/brother/sister." These comments are not helpful. What has happened to the child is the worst possible thing that could have happened at this moment, and it is best to be aware that trying to sugarcoat this in any way is not helpful.[11]

And if the child seems to feel left out or if they seem disengaged?

- Again, get them to help out. Allow the child to take an active part in the grief process and the rituals the family sets up for grieving.
- The child of this age likes to have a job. Let them hand out the programs at the funeral; let them pass around food at the wake; give them small jobs at home.
- Help the child to find creative ways to remember their lost loved one. Suggest doing a project: make a video or "story" out of photos on the phone or on social media, make a memory book or box, make some frames and put photos of the lost loved one in them.

It is important for children of this age to have a number of ways to express their feelings. Try to provide them with opportunities to talk, draw, or do other creative activities.

Children of this age also need help in figuring out what they want from their friends and their teachers at this time. Do they want to tell their friends what has happened themselves? Do they want a teacher or parent to do it?

If you are the parent of a child who has suffered a loss, with your child's knowledge, call the school and talk to the child's teacher and the school counselor or nurse about the bereavement and figure out how best to acknowledge this at school.

Children often appreciate subtle recognition of their loss from others. For a teacher who is not sure what to do, a parent or relative can suggest to the teacher that he or she say to the child in private, "I know your ____ died and that was very sad for you." Then the teacher can ask the child how she or he can help.

At home, it is important to keep routines and rules as consistent as possible, as with the younger child. If this is not possible:

- Talk to the child about changes before they happen.
- If you need to go away, even for a day, prepare the child ahead of time.
- Even for errands of several hours, tell them where you are going and when you will be back. Give them a way to get in touch with you while you are gone.
- Do whatever you can to provide the child of this age a sense of continuity and safety.

The Funeral

Many mental health experts feel that it is important that children be included in the funeral and other rituals commemorating the death of a loved one. Allowing the child to attend the funeral can be helpful as it allows her to truly recognize that the death has occurred. And she can see that she is one of many who share the sorrow of the loss. Moreover, at the funeral she may receive attention and support from relatives and friends.

But it is important for the parent or other adult to discuss attendance at the funeral with the child. The child needs to know what the funeral will be like, and then she can be asked if she would like to attend. Children as young as four or five are capable of making such a choice.

Explain to the child what a funeral is and what will happen there. One way to say this is to explain that a funeral is a way for everyone to say goodbye to the person who has died. The child can be told that very often we do not have an opportunity to say goodbye or to tell someone that we love them before they die, and the funeral is a way to do this. The child can be told that many people find funerals a good way to say goodbye, but some people find them much too sad and like to say goodbye in a different way.[12]

If it is customary in your family to have an open casket, ask your child if she would like to look in the casket or not. This is important as it can be very disturbing for children to see someone who is no longer alive. Never insist that the child go up to the casket or kiss the loved one in the casket.

It is also a very good idea for the child to be seated with a supportive adult during the service, particularly if she is under the age of ten. This adult can be there to comfort the child, to answer her questions, and even to go out and take a break if the child needs to.

A separate conversation can be held about going to the gravesite. You can tell children what will happen there and you can also ask them if they want to attend this part of the ceremony. Seeing the coffin of a loved one put into the ground is often excruciatingly painful for close loved ones—including the adults in the family—and it may be too much for some children. Going home after the funeral ceremony may be best for these children, while others may choose to go to the graveside. And some children, especially older children and teens, may even benefit from helping to fill the grave, as is the tradition in some religions.

Following the actual funeral, there are a variety of other rituals the child can be involved in. My clients often ask me if children should visit the cemetery in the months and years following the loss. Again, this is something to talk with the child about. It is important to explain that this is a way to remember their lost loved one. Some children prefer not to go, while others find it very helpful. Taking flowers, planting a tree, and other ways of taking care of the grave can allow the child to feel like she has something she can do for her lost loved one. Visiting the cemetery also works against the avoidance and denial of the death. Children may prefer to avoid being sad and mourning, but trips to the cemetery or to church or synagogue or mosque on days when their loved one is being remembered are ways to help them not to avoid these important feelings. These rituals allow a time and place for the expression of painful feelings and the sharing of memories. Many children will not be ready to take a trip to the cemetery in the weeks just after the loss, but at some point in their development they may actually ask to visit the loved one's grave and may want to make a tradition of doing so.

In the years to come, religious or cultural observances of the anniversary of the death can also help parents and their children share feelings about the death which might otherwise be difficult to bring up.

For example, in Judaism, a year after the death there is often a ceremony for what is called "the unveiling" of the gravestone. In the case of Matt's children aged eleven and fourteen, described earlier, the children were very clear that they did not want to go to the unveiling. Matt spoke with them about it, explaining who would be there and what would happen, and they each told him that they preferred not to go. Instead, they each spent the day with friends while their father and other family members attended the ceremony. Matt willingly accepted his children's choice and afterward he talked with them about what it had been like.

If you're a parent working with a therapist around what is best for your children following a loss, this will be a good place to explore how to handle your family's plans for funeral observances and the children's participation. Otherwise, parents may want to discuss this matter with a trusted friend, priest, pastor, rabbi, or imam. Other family members may not always be the best people with whom to discuss this as they may have strong opinions about what they think the children *should* do or even what they want the children to do.

In the absence of religious tradition or even in addition to religious observance, a family may want to create their own observances.

After the death or on the first anniversary of the death, the family might set up a table full of pictures of the lost loved one. Or, at some point, they might make a video collection of photos. Tech savvy children and teenagers may be especially adept at doing this and may want to be the ones to put a video together. With younger children, making or painting frames bought at a hobby shop to put pictures in can be a good activity, or they might want to help bake a special dessert or make a special meal to remember the loved one who has died. These sorts of observances can occur randomly, or they can be planned on the birthday of the lost loved one, or on Mother's Day or Father's Day for a parent who has died.

For many children—and even for teens—it can be very helpful to have ways of actively remembering their loved one who has died. While it is usually the case that children are left on their own to figure out how and whether to remember someone who has died, having activities, routines, and rituals for remembering can scaffold a child's or teen's developing ability to do so on their own.

I also recommend keeping photographs of the lost loved one displayed in the house and providing the children with their own copies to have in their rooms rather than hiding away pictures and other reminders as some families may be tempted to do, especially after a move or after a new partner has entered the family (in the case of the death of a parent).

Preteens (Eleven to Twelve Years Old)

Children at this age can sometimes act like teenagers and at other times they behave like younger children and want all the love and attention they received when they were small.

When a child of this age experiences the loss of a close loved one, the above will apply. They may seem like they are taking the news in stride or they may break down in tears and need a great deal of caretaking. Either way, they need explanations of what has happened suited to their age, and they also need an abundance of extra love and concern.

This will be true at home as well as at school.

Carmel Breathnach was eleven when her mother died of cancer. She has written extensively about her experience in her memoir *Briefly I Knew My Mother* and on her blog (see Resources, page 255). She describes how important teachers are for children who have experienced a loss, and she says that what helped her were kind, caring, and compassionate words from her teachers. She appreciated just being asked, "How are you doing today?" or "What would make you feel more comfortable in class today?" or "Would you like to sit by your friend today?" She also suggests providing grieving children with an option to leave class if they are having trouble concentrating or if they feel too sad. She suggests that schools have a designated quiet place where grieving children can go to draw or listen to music.[13]

One of the things Breathnach also mentions is that she wishes that one of the adults at her school had been assigned to check in with her each day in the weeks after her mother's death. As kind as some of her teachers were, she makes it clear that she really needed more support than she actually received.

At home, it is also important to provide extra love and attention for the child of this age, and at the same time to keep rules and routines as consistent as possible.

As with younger children, it can also be helpful to make sure to provide a role for children of this age in any grief rituals the family practices. The preteen is very capable and she can be given all sorts of jobs. If the family is sitting shiva or having a wake, she can help make food, pass food around, make the table look pretty, arrange the flowers, take the coats, or make a guest book. Preteens often like to help, and they feel better about themselves when they do. Again, taking an active role in their grief is preferable over a passive one.

Children of this age are also attuned to what is fair and what is not. They are often extremely vocal when they feel they have not been treated fairly. And when a parent, or close loved one dies, this is the most unfair event of all.

In brief, here is what you can do to help:

- **Make sure to keep the child in the loop about what has happened to their parent or close loved one.** Hold off on describing the most graphic details. As you know more, tell them more. Children of this age can be very perceptive, and they often want to know everything and be involved in whatever is going on.
- **Be prepared for an unusual reaction to the news.** Children of this age can have trouble controlling their emotional reactions, and they may later feel embarrassed about what they did when they heard about the death.[14]
- **Be prepared for the child of this age to be angry.** Their reaction to loss may include irritability or anger. They may feel that life has treated them unfairly or even that the person who died has betrayed them.
- **Make sure to let them know well in advance about any further losses or changes that are forthcoming.** This could be a move, someone coming to live in the home or leaving the home, or travel.
- **Over the coming weeks, be prepared for strong reactions to anything and everything.** But also be prepared for them to keep some—or even most—of their feelings private. Be aware that any drops in school performance may come about as a result of their sadness and preoccupation with their loss.
- **Be prepared for changes in attitude toward schoolwork or friends.** Some things that used to matter a great deal may not matter so much now, or some things that didn't matter at all before may matter more now.
- **Help the child reenter favorite activities.** If they want, go with them to the first sports practice or music lesson after their loss.
- **Encourage remembering the loved one who has died.** Look at pictures together, tell stories.

The Teen Years (Thirteen to Twenty)

Teenagers can be quite independent and self-sufficient. They may seem as though they do not want or need extra help with their grief when they lose a loved one.

However, nothing could be further than the truth.

Teenagers may want to seem self-sufficient but often they haven't a clue about how to feel or how to behave following a loss.

This was certainly true for me.

As I have described, I was quite frozen following my father's death. I did not cry much, and I leapt into action taking care of things around the house and trying to care for my mother.

But I did not know how to feel my own feelings. I buried them— or they buried themselves. I did not know how to deal with the fact that my father had died; I did not know how to talk to my friends or my teachers about it, and in my family, well, we just didn't talk about it.

This left me all alone with my experience. I felt like I just had to move ahead with life. Or, as my young friend Lucine said, I knew there were feelings, but they were "at a distance, across the road."

So, as a family member of a teen who has experienced a loss, or as a friend, it is important to pay special attention to the teen even if they appear independent and self-sufficient. And this applies not just to the week or two after the loss, but for the next several years.

During this time, the teen will be struggling with how to process their loss, how to integrate it into their life, how to feel, and how to let others know how they are feeling.

However, it is important to be careful in how you go about providing help. Teenagers are keen observers of adults, and they are often sensitive to any sign of condescension. Usually they want to be treated as competent, mature people at the very same time as they are desperate for help. They want to know that people care and are interested in how they feel—but they may also be quite private about their feelings.

If you have a teen, go forth cautiously:

- Ask how she is doing.
- Invite her to do an activity or have a meal together.
- See what she talks about and whether you can pick up on any clues about difficulties with feelings, friends, or focusing on schoolwork.
- Try not to make suggestions or give advice.
- Listen.
- And, if she seems to want it, offer up your own experiences with loss.

If you are the surviving parent in a family where the other parent has died, also consider the following:

- Make a point of asking your teen directly how she is doing. She may shrug, she may not answer, or she may react in a number of other ways, but don't let this put you off. And definitely, do not take this personally.
- Wait a few days and ask again. She needs to know that you are interested and that you are paying attention.
- Try spending some time together. Even if your teen does not acknowledge this directly, this kind of attention can be very, very important to her.

And the advice I have given for younger children especially holds true for teenagers. It is important to keep rules and routines as consistent as possible. When things change less, rather than more, this helps the teenager feel a sense of safety and security during a time when they are not sure that they can trust life, their own surroundings, or even their own feelings.

- If she had a curfew before, keep the curfew in place.
- If you need to rely on her to do more for you, let her know exactly what you need her to do. Helping out makes some teens feel a sense of purpose after a loss.
- Be sure to show your appreciation for what she is doing. But let the teen know that the same rules that used to apply still apply. Even if she is having to do some adult things, she is still a teenager and needs the rules and limits that teenagers usually have.
- Ask her if she wants help letting the other kids at school know that she has lost a loved one. If so, call the advisory teacher and ask them to speak to the class before the teen returns to school. It is helpful if the teacher can inform the class about what has happened in a brief and factual way and then suggest that the teen's friends talk to her normally and *not* be afraid to say, "I'm sorry your ____ died." This sort of direct intervention by the school can cut down on the circulation of rumors as well as on the awkwardness that may occur when the teen returns to school.

If you are a relative or close friend of a teen who has suffered a loss:

- Stay in touch.
- Initiate contact.
- Take the teen out to do some things you know she has interest in, no matter how simple. Get lunch. Go shopping. Go to the movies or the batting cages or a museum or just for a walk with the dog.
- Provide the teen with time to talk. And even if she seems to be on her phone the entire time, don't lose heart, you are still providing the opportunity for conversation should she choose to make use of it. Don't take this personally and don't stop inviting the teen to do things with you.

If you are the parent of a child who has had a loss, I hope the ideas included in this chapter will be of some help to you. And if you are a relative or friend of the family, remember, there are many ways to be of help to a child or a family who has suffered a loss. While it is natural to consider holding back, to think that giving the family their privacy is respectful, often feeling this way has to do with our own feelings of awkwardness around the subject of loss. Try to reach out. Try to offer whatever help or assistance you have to give.

CHAPTER 8

How to Help Children with Specific Types of Loss

There are many kinds of loss, each with its own particular difficulties. In this chapter, I will talk about children and teens who have lost a parent, those who have lost a grandparent or a sibling, and those who have suffered a loss due to war, illness, violence, or suicide.

How to Help a Child Whose Parent Has Died

If you are the parent of a child whose parent has died, you will likely be in deep grief yourself. As you read earlier, it is crucial for you to allow space for your own grief as this will help you to be available to your children (chapter 6, page 127).

This will be a horrible time for all of you—and all you can do to begin with is to survive and put one foot in front of the other.

Nothing can remove the pain of loss for you or for your child or teenager.

But some things *can* be done to help your child as she navigates the new terrain of loss.

First of all, a child who has lost a parent will often feel starved for attention. Anything that she received from the parent who died is now unavailable. And she may feel that there is no hope for retrieving that attention in the future.

If you are the parent of a child who has lost their other parent, or if you are a close relative or friend, here are some concrete things you can do:

Communicate with the child.

When a child's parent dies, tell her promptly what has happened. If possible, it is best if the other parent can provide this news. Give the child the details she wants to know—but only to the extent appropriate to her age and stage of development.

Tell her what will happen next—who will be caring for her, who will be visiting, and so on. Even the smallest of children need to be prepared for what is going to happen.

Keep her informed. This includes preparing her for what the funeral and other events will be like.

After the initial conversation about what happened, initiate frequent contact with your child; don't wait for the child to come to you. Provide space for conversations and for cuddles; go into her bedroom if she is spending a great deal of time there. Be respectful, but also push for more contact rather than less.

And don't shy away from talking about the parent who died. Don't be afraid that you will cause her to be sad by doing this. She is already sad. The loss of her parent will be forefront in the child's mind, no matter what her age, in the weeks and months after the loss. As we've discussed before, share with the child how you're feeling too.

Ask how the child is doing. Ask how it's going with friends.

Once she's back to school, ask how it is going there and whether it feels different to be at school now. But be sensitive—if the child does not respond, back off for a little while, move on to other subjects.

Continue to make contact and ask questions as the weeks and months go by. It is difficult to know when and what to ask, if you are being too intrusive or not attentive enough. But keep trying—and make sure to read your child's cues as you go to figure out whether to ask more or to relax your curiosity.

Notice if your child is seeing friends less, if her grades drop, or if she seems less interested in things she used to do. Notice if she is spending more time on social media or video games. Ask gently about these things. And don't shy away from asking directly if she thinks being sad is getting in the way of doing things she used to enjoy.

If you start dating again, let the child know, if you think this will be helpful. But wait to introduce the child to anyone you are seeing until you know that this is someone you are going to want in your life for a while. Be gentle with the introduction. Take it slow. Have the child meet the new person in your life for the first time outside of the home, perhaps doing a shared activity. And be sure to let the child know that no one will ever replace her parent. Be prepared for pushback—and try to be patient with this. Your child may feel loyal to her lost parent.

Prepare for your child to have periods when she does not seem sad.

Be prepared for your child to seem to pop in and out of grief.[1] Children and teens do not mourn the same way that adults do, and for many children, sadness may alternate with periods during which they play and go back to their old activities.

If you have a teenager, be prepared for her to withdraw and/or to be irritable. These may be the ways she shows her upset over loss. Be patient—try not to react immediately to her moodiness or harsh comments. Take some time before you respond to her in order to avoid too many arguments. Try to make sure she spends some time with others—especially at mealtimes. And do not hesitate to ask her to help out around the house. Having specific jobs to do may help her to feel better about herself and may provide her with a sense of purpose. But of course, this does not mean that she won't complain about any work you ask her to do!

Make your home a comforting place by keeping mealtimes and bedtimes consistent as much as possible. Offer favorite foods for a few weeks. Don't worry about serving pizza too often. Be flexible about where everyone sleeps for a while.

Be observant.

Your child or teen may seem uncooperative, she may misbehave or refuse to do what you want her to do. At this point, much of what you are seeing will be her reaction to loss.

After the first few weeks, if your child or teen is still withdrawn socially, offer to accompany her to activities and/or encourage her to see friends.

After a few months, if your child or teen is still irritable, misbehaving, or withdrawn, talk to her about what you notice. Start slowly and be kind. You can say something as simple as "I've noticed you've stayed in your room more recently" or "I've noticed that you've seemed unhappy recently." Again, don't hesitate to ask if she thinks this is because she's been so sad or so upset about her loss.

Ask her what she think could help. And don't refrain from asking if she would like to talk to a grief counselor or therapist or join a group.

Be present.

Spend time with your child to the extent that you are able.

Provide extra attention and affection. Especially in the first weeks and months after your child's parent has died, time spent together will be precious to your child and valuable to her as she moves forward in her grief. Remember, she may feel very alone.

Prepare for back-to-school.

Ask your child or teen when she will be ready to go back to school. Allow at least a few days for her to mourn and be at home—but probably not more than a week.

Speak with your child about how she would like her classmates to learn about her loss. With that information in hand, either speak to the school's principal and classroom teacher and let them know what has happened or help your child to figure out what she will say herself.

Help your child transition back to school. Ask if she wants you to accompany her into the building the first day back.

Seek out the resources you need.

If your child is still very anxious or depressed for more than one to three months after her loss, inquire gently whether she might like to talk to a grief counselor or a therapist.

To find one, ask trusted friends, ask your pediatrician, or look on the *Psychology Today* website (https://www.psychologytoday.com/us /therapists), which has profiles of people in your area.

Find additional resources in your community for children who have lost a parent. Ask your child whether she would like to attend any of these, whether they are grief groups, gatherings at a grief center, or a summer camp for kids who have lost a parent. Getting to know other children or teens who have lost a parent can help a bereaved child to feel less alone.

Don't hesitate to find a grief counselor or therapist for yourself. Losing a partner or coparent is very, very hard. Being a solo parent is hard. Being a parent while grieving is hard. Knowing what to say and how to handle your child after such an enormous loss is hard. Do not be afraid to reach out. Talking to someone can help you to be more available for your child and to provide them with what they need during this time.

Create opportunities to remember your loved one.

In the coming years, provide opportunities for mourning and remembering.

- Offer to take the child or teen to the graveyard if that is comfortable for you.

- On holidays, develop some family rituals for remembering the lost parent.[2]
- Keep framed photos of the lost parent up or give your child some to keep in her room.

Help the child as she continues to revise her internal idea of who her parent was. She will work on this over the years. Reevaluating her parent as she gets older will be part of this. Hearing the stories and memories of others will also be a part of this. Listen to her as she works on this—and resist the temptation to tell her what she should think or how you think she should remember her parent.

How to Help a Child Whose Sibling Has Died

If you are the parent of a child who has died, you will be in deep grief and mourning. Taking time for your own feelings and your own grief will need to be a top priority for you.

But the cruel reality is that at the same time as you need to do this, your other children will also need you. They have also suffered a terrible loss.

Let me offer some recommendations.

Put time aside for yourself.

Try to put some time aside for yourself. Bringing in extra childcare may be necessary at this time.

But also try to be available to your children for at least some time each day. Try your best to watch and listen to them in order to find out how they are feeling and what their reaction is to the loss of their sibling. Try to get yourself to talk with them about what happened, about how you feel and about their feelings. And most of all, remind them how much you love them. This may be hard for you to feel at this time—you may be thinking mostly of the child you no longer have—but do your best to let your children know that they are of the utmost importance to you.

Acknowledge the child's loss.

Children and teens who have lost a sibling desperately need validation that not only their parents but they themselves have suffered a grievous loss. Elizabeth DeVita-Raeburn writes about this in her memoir *The Empty Room* in which she describes what it was like after her brother died. She writes about how rare it was for anyone to acknowledge her loss after her brother's death and how common it was for everyone to focus on her parents and how she needed to help them out.

For her book she also interviewed other children who lost a sibling and found that it was very important to them when people spoke to them about their feelings or sent a condolence letter addressed just to them.[3]

So if you are the parent of a child who has lost a sibling, make sure you acknowledge to your child that she has also suffered a huge loss—and that you are *both* sad about this. Try to emphasize that you are in this together—even though this may be very hard for you at this point.

Grief can be a world unto itself, and it is easy to feel like retreating into it by yourself. But, again, try to spend some time each day communicating with your partner and your children.

And if you are an adult who is close to the family and if you are offering condolences to the parents of a child who has died, make a point of also speaking to the children in the family about how sorry you are that they have lost a brother or sister.

If you are writing a condolence letter, consider writing more than one—one for the parents and one for each child in the family.

Ask the child about their experience.

If you are the parent, grandparent, aunt, uncle, or close friend of a child whose sibling has died, and if the child seems to want to talk, ask them about their own experience. Don't focus on their parents. Feel free to talk about your own losses—even if you are much older than they. Children who have suffered a loss both have their own unique set of experiences and feelings and they are looking for a road map. How should they feel? What should they do? Be alert to signs that they want to hear more—or less—about your experience of loss.

Help the child to fill their time and create new routines.

Another thing you can do to help a child who has lost a sibling is to help them to create new routines and rituals in their lives—whether to commemorate their sibling or simply to establish new patterns and habits for themselves. It will be hard for them to learn how to live without their brother or sister. Especially in the weeks and months right after the death, offer to help them fill their free time. Even the simplest of errands or activities can be comforting. Being at home may be especially painful for a child with all the emptiness that is left by a sibling who has died.

Remind the child that their parents love them.

And finally, whether you are a grandparent, aunt, uncle, or friend, one of the most important things you can do for a child or teen who has lost a sibling is to remind them that their parents love them and always have.

As mentioned, a child or teen who loses a sibling can often feel that all the attention being paid to the loss is evidence that the child who died was and is loved more than they are. This conclusion is almost universal, and children need to be reminded—frequently—that when someone dies, a *lot* of attention is paid to their death and to mourning them—but that this does not mean that the child who died was loved more than the other children in the family who are still alive.

You can say, quite simply, "You know your mother and father are spending all their time thinking and talking about your brother/sister right now. And that is because of what has happened. It is because they've died. But it is not because they loved your brother/sister more than you. They love you too and they always will."

How to Help a Child Whose Grandparent Has Died

When a child's grandparent dies, like when a sibling dies, so much of the attention goes to the parent whose parent died.

And if you are the parent whose parent has died, you will be having many feelings of your own right now—and you will be needing extra attention or nurturing sent your way. You will also need time for yourself.

Again, let me offer some recommendations.

Ask for help.

So, as mentioned previously, do not hesitate to bring in help—a beloved nanny or an aunt or a grandparent from the other side of the family may be able to help by doing more childcare right now and by providing extra love and attention for your children.

At the same time, it is also important for you to try to address your child's or children's feelings, concerns, and questions as best you can. Your children will want to know how their grandparent died, why they died now, and how to feel and behave. If this is the first time they have experienced a death, they may also have lots of questions about death in general.

Be there for the child.

If you are an adult who is close to a child whose grandparent has died, try to be there for the child (or children). Try spending extra time with the child while the parents have time to themselves. It will be helpful to the child who has lost a grandparent to get to talk about their feelings. It will also be helpful for them to feel useful.

Find ways for the child to help.

Doing something with the child to help them to feel useful may be especially appreciated. Offer to help them bake a special treat for their parent, or make a frame to put a picture of their grandparent in. Or perhaps they would like to tell you some stories about their grandparent.

If there is a funeral or memorial service, perhaps you can offer to sit near the child and be available to take her out for a break during the service if she should want this.

In the weeks and months after the grandparent has died, don't forget that the child is still mourning, and there may still be an absence in the child's life. That absence may have come about as a result of the loss of the grandparent, if they were close, or it may have come about because their parent is preoccupied with their own mourning. The child may need others to fill in that space with extra love and attention.

How to Help Children Who Have Experienced Loss Associated With Violence

In today's world, children are exposed to violence on a daily basis—through the video games they play, the news they see on TV or in the newsfeeds on their phones, walking down the street or in their very schools. Violence is everywhere for many children.

We don't like to acknowledge this. We prefer to downplay the importance of the violence in the movies kids are watching or the content of the video games they are playing. We don't like to think of how violent some neighborhoods are or how likely a local shooting or a school shooting may be. But uncomfortable as it is to acknowledge, viewing violence and being exposed to violence affects children in an extremely negative way.

Studies demonstrate that children exposed to violent media may become numb to violence, they may imitate the violence, and they may show more aggressive behavior. Younger children and those with emotional, behavioral, or learning problems may be even more influenced by violent images than other children.[4]

So in and of itself, exposure to violent news, violent videos, violent social media, and violent video game content presents difficulty for children and teens and represents a multitude of losses for these kids. Children and teens exposed to violence potentially lose a sense of calm, safety, and security, some may lose trust in their world, some may lose their ability to focus and concentrate, some may experience increased difficulty controlling themselves or their own emotions, and some may be traumatized.

Here are a few things you can do to help children limit their exposure to violence in the media:

- Avoid having the television news on when children under the age of twelve are in the room.
- Restrict children's use of social media and newsfeeds prior to the age of twelve.
- Choose which platforms you allow your child under twelve to use.
- Talk to teens over the age of twelve about what they are seeing on their social media, on video games, and in movies. Try not

to argue or lecture. Ask them what they think about what they are seeing and how they think it affects them and their friends.

Exposure to actual violence is of course even worse than exposure to violence via the screen.

Children who experience violence in their homes, in their neighborhoods, in their schools, or in their countries are at risk in innumerable ways. Their sense of trust in the world as a safe place is inevitably damaged, and their ability to rely on their parents and the institutions they are part of to protect them is interfered with.

Research has shown that children who are exposed to and who experience violence develop more physical and emotional difficulties as a result of the stress they experience.

The most well-known research in this area is known as the ACE study (ACE standing for Adverse Childhood Events). It was conducted by the Centers for Disease Control and Kaiser Permanente in the mid-1990s with a group of patients insured through Kaiser Permanente, and subsequent studies on inner-city children expanded on the original findings. The initial study focused on how traumatic childhood events may negatively affect adult health. It was found that toxic stress from ACEs can negatively affect children's brain development, immune systems, and stress-response systems and that these changes can affect children's attention, decision-making, and learning. Children growing up with toxic stress may have difficulty forming healthy and stable relationships. It was found that there is a direct link between childhood trauma and adult onset of chronic disease, incarceration, and employment challenges, with the higher number of ACEs resulting in greater incidence of negative outcomes.[5]

So, exposure to violence is overwhelming, it is damaging, and it is traumatic. But there may be some things you can do:

- Maintain your own home as a safe space for your children to the extent that you are able. Do this by keeping all unsecured

weapons out of the home and by insisting on keeping inter-
personal conflict at the lowest level possible.

- Try to establish as much stability within your home as possible. Do this by keeping rules and routines as constant as you
  can. Set limits with your children and teens and follow
  through. Flexibility is sometimes necessary, but remember,
  many studies have shown that children and teens feel safest
  when rules are consistent.

- If you feel you need a firearm for the protection of your family, always keep any firearms in your home under lock and
  key. There are no exceptions to this rule. Keep all ammuni-
  tion stored in a separate location, also under lock and key.
  Educate your children about firearms and their appropriate
  use. Let your children know that any guns you own are only
  there for the protection of the home and they will never be
  used for any other purpose. Set clear rules and boundaries—
  for example, you can say, "If you see a gun, tell me. Do not
  touch it. No matter how curious you are about it, come to
  me." And set consequences for contact with firearms for children and teens. For example, you can say, "Under no circumstances are you to touch or possess a gun. If you do, the
  consequence will be ____." (Add your own consequence here,
  but make sure it is extremely strict.) Let your children know
  exactly how unsafe it is for them to touch or hold a gun.

- Frequently remind your children that you are trying to keep
  them as safe as you possibly can.

- Consider supporting antiviolence initiatives or similar community organizations that are important to you.

When violence does strike, and when it results in the loss of a
friend or acquaintance, a community member, or especially when it
results in the loss of a child's loved one, the child who is affected is at
tremendous risk.

The likelihood that difficulties will arise in their mourning and recovery processes and in their overall development is high.

According to the Trauma and Grief Center (TAG) at Children's Hospital New Orleans, when a child loses a loved one to violence, it can permanently change their world view, making them believe that the world is a scary and dangerous place. If a child's mother is the victim of violence, for instance, common preoccupying thoughts can include "If this can happen to my mom, it can happen to anybody" or "Nobody can keep me safe."

In part 1, I spoke about the teenagers who experienced the loss of friends and schoolmates in Uvalde, Texas, and Parkland, Florida, and about Brenda Valenzuela, who watched as her teacher and nine of her classmates were shot at her community college. These are children, teens, and young adults whose world view has been changed forever and who will suffer the aftereffects of exposure to extreme violence for their entire lives.

Like the survivors of school shootings, many of the children seen at the TAG Center in New Orleans who have experienced losses due to violence and who have experienced violence in their neighborhoods are scared to step outside their homes. Some are afraid to go to school for fear that something might happen to them on their way there or while they are there. Some feel uncomfortable playing in the park because they are afraid of being shot. Many of the children and adolescents treated there have given up on their hopes and dreams for the future.

These children and teens need a great deal of help with all these feelings.

Of course, everything mentioned so far about how to help bereaved children will be relevant to them, but the following recommendations will also be especially important.

If you know or have a child or teen who has experienced a loss due to violence, whether at school, in the community, at home, or even in the media when a public figure or beloved singer or sports star dies due to a violent act, do not avoid talking about it. Start right away and try the following:

- **Acknowledge what has happened in conversations with the child.** It is hard to talk about loss, especially if it happened in a particularly violent way, but the reality is that the child has experienced something extremely difficult and she needs to know that it is okay to talk about it.[6]
- **Minimize exposure to the media.** If the child's loss is portrayed in the media—for example, in the case of a school shooting or a murder—turn off the TV news and, if you are the parent, ask to keep your child's phone for several days or encourage her to stay away from social media and her newsfeeds. Let her know that seeing and reading about what has happened can be retraumatizing for her and may only make her feel more overwhelmed and more upset.[7]
- **Provide a sense of safety and security.** The most important thing caregivers can do for their children is to remind them that the adults in their lives are doing everything they can to keep them safe and protected.[8] If you can, and if she wants or needs you to, accompany your child to school or to after-school activities until she feels safe enough to go on her own again.
- **Be proactive and know the signs of trauma.** Among pre-school-age children, look out for significant regressions such as language delays, toileting accidents, bed-wetting, difficulties sleeping, repeating nightmares, changes in eating patterns, or excessive clinginess with caregivers. In older school-age children, signs of trauma may include avoidance of activities they once enjoyed, irritability or aggressive behavior, bed-wetting, new fears and anxieties, recurrent nightmares and intrusive images, or engaging in risk-taking behaviors.[9] And in teens, signs of trauma include significant regressions,

withdrawal from friends and/or family, intrusive thoughts, repeating nightmares, flashbacks, intense anxiety, severe depression, risky behavior, and suicidality.

- **Know what resources you have.** Seek out professional help for your child or yourself as soon as you can following the loss. This may include group therapy or individual therapy and/or consulting with your child's school counselor. Read more about this in chapter 9.
- **Embrace community.** Bring in all the resources you can, including your spiritual community, your extended family, and your school community to provide extra support for you and your child. Become a part of at least one caring community, and encourage your child to participate with you.

Remember that every child is different, experiences are not identical, and the needs of each child, family, and community will vary.

But in all cases, children who have experienced loss due to violence have suffered a double trauma and a double loss. They have been exposed to something terrible and frightening *and* they have lost a loved one. They will need a great deal of love, support, and help to proceed with their mourning, their development, and their lives.

How to Help a Child Who Has Experienced the Suicide of a Loved One

The loss of a loved one through suicide is a deeply troubling event for anyone of any age. It is shocking and disturbing. Questions are inevitable. Why did my loved one do this? Did I do anything to cause this? Or is there something I could have done to prevent it?

These questions are torturous. They don't have definitive answers. Often, they last a lifetime.

And for children and teenagers, all of these things are especially true.

For the youngest of children, ages one through three, suicide will be a difficult concept to understand. At this age it may be better to postpone the actual mention of suicide, and it may be sufficient to talk to the child about the fact that the person has died.

Eventually, however, even young children of this age may overhear others talking and they may hear the word suicide, or they might hear about what the person did to themselves. At this point, they may be confused, and it will be important to explain in the simplest terms what has happened and why.

Starting at around age four or five, the age at which a child can understand the concept of suicide, a discussion is necessary as soon as the death has occurred.

Be honest.

First, it is important to be honest. The explanation that you give can be suited to their age and stage of development, and it does not need to be explicit, but it should not be inaccurate.

So, to the curious four-year-old who asks what happened to the person who died by suicide, a simple explanation can be given.

For example, a parent can say, "Uncle Tom was very, very unhappy for a very, very long time and he didn't feel that anyone could help him. We tried, the doctors tried, his friends tried, but finally he just did not want to live anymore—so he made sure that he would die."

For a child capable of understanding a little more, you can talk about what was bothering the person who died by suicide. From age six and up, children can understand about depression or psychosis if an appropriate explanation is given.

You can say something like, "Daddy had an illness called depression (or psychosis). This made him think things that weren't true. And it made him feel that he should die. I tried to help him as well as I could—and he did love me and he did love you—but his illness was just too strong."

Answer questions.

But be prepared—more questions will be forthcoming.

Children may want to know about how the person killed himself. And whether you answer this question will be a matter of discretion. Do you think the child can manage the facts? If not, it can suffice to say to them that you will tell them when they are a bit older. You can add that it is very sad and difficult to talk about. However, if you think that there is any chance that your child will hear about how their loved one died from someone else, or if you think they may over-hear conversations, it is better for you to tell them the truth, even if you are not sure if they are ready to hear it. It is always better for this information to come directly from a parent or very close loved one. But this is an extremely difficult conversation for most parents to have with a child. So let me provide some ideas.

First, be aware that your child will think deeply about the details you provide. You want to tell the truth while also trying to not provide details that will be overly troubling. Choose your words carefully.

For a teenager, you will be best just telling her directly what happened. If the loved one was depressed or psychotic, be sure to talk about this and of course mention that if the teen herself ever feels depressed or has thoughts she feels she cannot control, you will be there to help and you will want the teen to tell you about this rather than trying to hurt or kill herself.

If the loved one shot himself, you can say, "Uncle Tom used a gun to kill himself. And this is something that no one should ever do. There were many ways that Uncle Tom could have gotten help for himself, and we all wished that he had. We are all devastated and wish we could have done more for him." Use your own words, but do not be afraid to go into detail about how deeply sad and disturbing this is to you.

If the child's loved one crashed their car on purpose, this is something you can also tell your child or teen, and in this case, you will still want to say that this is something that no one should ever do, that it is dangerous not only for the person driving but for other people on the road, and that this is also against the law.

For a parent whose family member has died by suicide, there is always the fear that the children or teens in the family will be influenced by what has happened and may, at some point, want to kill themselves in the same way—or in a similar way—to that of the loved one. This is terrifying, but it is not a reason to refrain from talking about what has happened, In fact, talking about it and expressing your own horror and upset and sadness about the suicide can provide an important message to your child or teen that suicide is an event that deeply injures the loved ones of the person who has died.

Be reassuring.

After hearing about a suicide, children and teens may become anxious about whether other people they know or love could do the same thing—or even whether they themselves might ever feel like killing themselves.

It is important to talk to children about these feelings and to acknowledge that it is scary when someone takes their own life. But it is also important to reassure the child or teen as often as necessary that most people can be helped to feel better when they feel upset or hopeless, that talking to friends and relatives is usually very helpful, and even when it is not, that doctors and therapists have many ways to help. Call the illness that the loved one suffered from by name. You can say, "Depression is very hard to live with" or "There are good medicines for psychosis and someone can usually feel better with the right treatment."

Counteract feelings of self-blame.

It is also of the utmost importance to talk to children about any feelings of self-blame that they may have. Even if they do not bring up feeling responsible for the person's suicide, you can say, "After someone kills themself, people who loved them often wonder if there was something they could have done to help the person while they were alive. They also sometimes wonder if they did something to cause the person to want to die. But nothing I did and nothing you did caused this and there was nothing we could have done to prevent it—even though we wish we could have."

The suicide of a loved one is one of the most devastating losses a child can suffer. It is different in so many ways from loss due to illness or accident, even a loss due to violence, because in the case of suicide there is intentionality—the person who died chose to die. This leaves all those who cared for the person in a permanent kind of limbo, wondering exactly why this happened and wishing they could have done more.

Children who perseverate on the loss or the manner of loss, who seem to be thinking a great deal about it even weeks after the event, may need some professional help. They may need to see a therapist to process this loss as well as to understand better about suicide.

Children or teens who seemed genuinely depressed after the suicide of a loved one, especially in the case of the loss of a parent, a beloved relative, or a boyfriend or girlfriend, must be watched carefully at home and seen by a professional as soon as possible. It is sometimes the case, especially in older children and in teens, that the child may be considering suicide themself.

In the following chapter, I will discuss the options available for treatment.

CHAPTER 9

Professional Treatment Options

Some adults and some children will respond to a significant loss with the expected and normal processes of sadness, grief, and mourning. They may need the support of friends and loved ones but not require any professional help at all.

Others may experience their bereavement as particularly difficult and disorganizing.[1] In this case, an experienced therapist can be very helpful.

A therapist can evaluate whether an adult or child is experiencing difficulty in progressing in their grief process, whether their mourning has gone awry, and to what extent they need help to get back on course.

For more advice on seeking professional help as an adult, refer back to chapter 4.

If a child has experienced loss and is not moving ahead with her grieving process, if you see signs that she is stuck in her sadness or her anger, if she has become withdrawn or seems numb, if she has expressed the desire to stop living, or if you see signs that she is not doing well in any way, you may consider taking her for therapy.

Perhaps you feel that the way you and others in the child's life have tried to help has not succeeded, or perhaps you notice signs that the child is not doing well. You may observe that the child is having trouble falling asleep at night or that she is having reoccurring nightmares. Perhaps she is not seeing her friends as much as she used to. Maybe she is not eating—or she is eating more than usual. Or maybe her grades have dropped.

All of these can be signs of difficulty. And if it has been three to six months since the child's loss, these can be signs that professional help could be useful.

But most importantly, if you, as a parent, think your child may need therapy, that is reason enough to seek out help.

If you are not sure if your child needs professional help, check this list. If any one or more of these apply to your child, consider seeking therapy for her:

1. You fear that the child's loss was truly traumatic for her.
2. You see treatment as a way to prevent future difficulties for her.
3. As a parent of the child, you feel that you are not sufficiently available to her, perhaps because of your own mourning process.
4. The death the child has been affected by occurred by suicide.
5. There was a very poor relationship between the child and the loved one who died.
6. In the case of the loss of a parent, there is a very poor relationship between child and the surviving parent or that parent suffers from a mental illness.
7. The lost loved one was mentally ill and living with the family the year prior to their death.
8. The child is a girl who lost her mother and she is under the age of eighteen.
9. The child lost a parent and is under the age of four.
10. The child has suffered from anxiety or depression in the past.
11. The child is a boy and his father died during his teen years.
12. The child is a boy and his father or mother died from cancer of the reproductive organs.
13. The child is a girl and her mother died during or shortly after childbirth, or due to breast cancer, or her father or mother died from cancer of the reproductive organs.
14. The child has experienced severe economic hardship or a sudden move following the death and is showing signs that she is having trouble adapting to these changes.
15. The child has lost one or both parents, and there is no one available to take over her care.

16. The child has lost a parent, and the remaining parent shows signs of pathological mourning.
17. The remaining parent has increased physical intimacy with the child to an extent that seems inappropriate to the developmental needs of the child or is more related to the needs of the parent than the child.
18. The child does not cry in the first month after the death.
19. The child is over four and does not talk about a parent who has died or the fact of the parent's death.
20. The death was of a close loved one and was abrupt and unexpected.
21. The death resulted from a terminal illness that lasted more than six months and/or was unusually disfiguring or resulted in cognitive deterioration.
22. The family did not explain the illness or death to the child or deliberately concealed the illness or death from the child.
23. The family delayed informing the child of death when others knew for more than one day.

What Does Therapy Do?

In the play *Macbeth*, Shakespeare wrote, "Give sorrow words: the grief that does not speak whispers the o'erwrought heart and bids it break." I quoted this in the preface because it is so true—and so important to remember.

After the loss of a dear loved one, if a child cannot acknowledge her loss and put her feelings into words, or if she cannot show them in her play or in her artwork, she is at risk.

And this is true for adults as well.

Expressing feelings of confusion and sadness and sorrow and anger after loss is critical to recovery.

And if a bereaved child cannot do this, she is at risk for developing difficulty moving through her grief process and for continuing along in her healthy development. She is at risk for developing a long-lasting depression, for developing an anxiety disorder, for developing bodily symptoms, and for developing difficulties with relationships.

The poet and writer Natasha Trethewey said this about her experience after her mother's murder when she was nineteen, "If I had not been able to tell the story I ran the risk of being overtaken [by grief]. I had to put my grief in the mouth of language, because it's the only thing that will grieve with me."[2]

After a loss, some children and teens will understand what has happened, accept it and talk about it—while others seem to need more help to realize that the loss is real, to acknowledge it, and to express their thoughts and feelings about it.

Parents and family members can encourage the child or teen to talk about the loss, and they can model how to talk about it by doing so themselves. However, if they are not successful in helping the child or teen express her feelings, there are a number of options that may help.

A mental health provider who specializes in the treatment of grief and mourning can meet with the child or teen on a regular basis to talk with her and/or to play or do artwork with her to see if, together, they can begin to understand and put into words what the child or teen feels about her loss. Or the provider can do some behavioral exercises with the child or teen to work on better understanding and working through her grief.

There is quite of bit of research demonstrating that therapy can be very helpful both in treating existing distress due to loss and in preventing future symptoms.

Jessica Koblenz, a researcher who is interested in grief in childhood, wrote that research shows that bereaved children who have received treatment often do better than those who have not.[3]

She mentions the work of other researchers who found that individual or group therapy for bereaved children may reduce the risk of their developing anxiety and depression. Social skills training and relaxation training have also been found to be helpful in decreasing depressive symptoms for bereaved children.[4]

But how do you go about finding a therapist for your child?

The first and most important aspect of finding a therapist is locating someone who is both experienced with and attuned to the feelings and processes of grief.

It is important to find someone who comes well recommended, if possible. You may be able to find such a person by asking friends, relatives, your pediatrician, or your own doctor. You can also look on *Psychology Today*'s website to find a therapist who lists grief work with children as one of their specialties and then check what kind of ratings they have gotten. It is important to find someone with experience and sensitivity as providing psychotherapy to bereaved children and teens is a task requiring experience, training, and deep reservoirs of compassion. The therapist must know how to meet the child or teen where she is and to proceed at the child's pace. She must know both how to talk with children and how to not talk—to be able to play or do artwork together, or just to sit together.

But individual therapy for the child or teen is not the only option. Following a loss in the family, it can also be helpful for the parent to have someone to talk to for themselves or in some cases for the entire family to go into family therapy together.

In the following pages, I will go over the options for various forms of psychotherapy to choose from following a loss in the family.

Option 1: Psychotherapy for the Parent

If you and your child have suffered a loss and if you are feeling overwhelmed by your grief, it is important for you to get help for yourself.

Or if you are someone who knows a parent who is overwhelmed by her grief, or a parent who is severely traumatized by her experience of loss, or a parent who is finding it difficult to care for her children and to attend to their grief, it will be important to aid that parent in getting help for herself—and individual psychotherapy is one form of such help.

In individual psychotherapy, parents have a safe place to talk about all of their feelings. They will have an opportunity to grieve and to learn how to move through grief.

This individual therapy may focus only on the parent or it may also include helping the parent how to understand and aid the children in the family.

As mentioned, the best way to find a good therapist is through word of mouth. Ask others you know who have been in therapy whether they would recommend their therapist. You can also look for someone in your area who specializes in grief and loss, or you can call your local community mental health center or the Department of Psychiatry at the closest medical school. In-person therapy will be best if you can manage it, but therapy using an online platform may be more convenient. Be aware, however, that the large online therapy companies may not be the best place to look.

Option 2: Parental Guidance

Parental guidance is another option for parents of bereaved children that is different from individual therapy for the parent. It is a form of therapy during which a parent is able to learn about her children's feelings and behaviors rather than concentrating more on herself and her own feelings. This is a good choice when a parent is doing well handling her own grief but needs extra support in learning how to help her grieving child.

One of the first interventions a therapist may make in parental guidance is to help the parent to understand that her child neither experiences loss nor understands death in the same way as the parent.

The parent can then be helped to view the loss from the child's emotional· perspective.

In parental guidance, a therapist will help parents understand the limitations of the child's ability to understand death at her particular developmental level. The parent can then be helped to explain death to the child in a way that is appropriate to the child's level of understanding.

Through parental guidance, the parent can also be helped to become more comfortable talking about emotions and about expressing them with her child.

In some families, feelings are generally kept private and the expression of feelings is not customary. It may even be felt that demonstrations of love and attachment are only for babies and little children. In these families, it is extremely important that the parents, or in the case of the death of a parent, the surviving parent, understand that it is crucial for the child, no matter what her age, to be able to express her feelings—including her love for her lost loved one, her sadness, her anger, her confusion—*all* of her feelings!

Even in families where emotional expression is welcome, a child may be discouraged from fully experiencing and expressing her feelings because the parents may find it too difficult to see their child's pain or to be reminded of their own painful feelings.

Or, in some cases, the child herself may feel inhibited about expressing her feelings. She may feel that it will place an additional burden on her surviving parent and she may not want to do this. Or she may feel embarrassed about her feelings or shy about expressing them.

In these instances, a therapist providing parental guidance can explain how important the expression of feelings really is. This sometimes helps the parent who has come for parental guidance to then feel free to express her own feelings and to use the therapist as a container for these feelings. She can talk to the therapist about her own sadness, anger, fear, or overwhelm. In doing this, the parent may come to better accept both her own feelings and those of her child.

And sometimes, when a parent feels more able to express feelings, their child may also be able to feel freer to express feelings.

Susan Coates studied parents who lost their spouses at the World Trade Center on 9/11. She found that parents often sought treatment for their children and not for themselves even though they were experiencing significant difficulty overcoming the trauma of 9/11 and the loss of their partner.[5]

If you have lost your spouse, it can feel overwhelming. But with time you may be able to understand that life will go on. In parental guidance, the therapist helps the parent understand that for the child, the loss of a parent, especially early in life, is different. There will never be another mother or father for the child. This is a loss like no other.

I gained insight into this when I asked a colleague what it had been like to lose his mother at the age of three.

He explained to me that, as a three-year-old boy, it had felt as though, in adult terms, his wife had died, all of his children had died, his house had burned down, he had lost his job, and he had lost all of his friends and his means of communicating.

He said that the loss of his mother at that age had been totally overwhelming and had sent him into a state of complete confusion and anxiety.[6]

This is the sort of explanation that the parent of a young child may need to hear in order to fully understand their child's experience of loss.

When parents do not understand their child's experience, this can increase the child's distress. As Susan Coates said about the widows and widowers of 9/11, "Where parents were unable to take in and keep in mind what their children were experiencing, children seemed to develop more stress related symptoms, to struggle more with states of shut down and confusion, and perhaps transiently to feel unable to know what was real."[7]

Contrary to popular belief, some specific details about the illness or the accident that caused the death can be provided for children of all ages. A therapist can help with what to say and how to say it.

Parental Guidance in Special Circumstances

For families in which one parent is terminally ill, the therapist providing parental guidance to the well parent may recommend bringing in the child for a few sessions—and even including the ill parent if they are able to participate. Although it is difficult to consider doing this, it can be very helpful for everyone to talk about what is happening at present and what will happen when the ill parent dies. The therapist can help both of the parents and the child to prepare for the inevitable decline and loss of the parent who is ill. The ill parent can talk about what she wants for her partner and her child after she is gone.

In future sessions, the therapist can help the well parent to figure out how to keep the child informed about what is happening, what is likely to happen. and to guide the child as to the best ways to express her feelings to her ill parent.

In the case of a violent or potentially traumatizing death, parental guidance can help parents to decide how to talk with the child about what has happened. Susan Coates outlined steps that can be taken to help in this situation.

First, the parent can be reassured about their own reactions. It is important for them to know that even extreme reactions to a violent or shocking event do not mean they are going crazy and that their fears, anxieties, and flashbacks are normal reactions to a severely traumatizing event.

Second, the parent can be helped to understand their child's reactions to the event—especially if the parent finds it odd or perplexing. Coates helped parents who had lost a partner on 9/11 to understand their children's drawings, dramatic play, dreams, nightmares, and fantasies. And this helped the parents begin to be able to reflect more productively on their child's experience.

Third, the parent can be helped to further understand the child's experience. Coates found that some parents became angry or disturbed by their children's increased clinginess, anger, or tantrums. Parents were afraid that these reactions were signs of lasting damage or future pathology. She helped parents to see these as expectable and temporary responses.

Coates points out that therapists can also help parents to see the importance of protecting children from adult conversations about the event. And the parents can be helped to see the value in having the family return to normal routines as soon as possible.

Option 3: Joint Therapy of the Parent and Child

If both you and your child are grieving, another option for therapy is treatment that includes your child in the room with you. This is particularly useful if the child is under five years old. Small children are especially close to their parents, and they will often pick up on their parent's feelings and take cues from their parent as to how to feel themselves.

Another important reason to have therapy together is that children and parents who have been traumatized by the same event may have lost touch with one another's feelings due to their preoccupation with their own pain and devastation. Joint treatment can be used to renew a close relationship and to understand each other in a deep way.

In her work with children who lost a parent on 9/11, Susan Coates noticed just this. In many cases, the trauma of 9/11 affected the children's relationship with their surviving parent. She found that while some relationships helped to protect against traumatization for the child, in other cases traumatization worked to put both parents and children out of touch with each other.[8] This observation is extremely important because the bereaved child needs an untraumatized, emotionally available surviving parent to help them with their feelings.

In joint therapy, the parent, the child, and the therapist often do a shared activity. They may play a game or participate in imaginative play. The therapist then has the opportunity to see how engaged the parent and child are with each other, where miscommunications may occur, and what feelings each has toward the other. The therapist can talk to them both in ways that they both understand about what they may be feeling.

So, joint therapy can help both the parent and the child to mourn, it can help each understand the feelings of the other, and it can rebuild the attachment and security so important for both parent and child after a significant loss.

Option 4: Individual Therapy for the Child

Sometimes, parental guidance or joint therapy is not the best choice. In some cases, individual therapy for the parent and/or for the child will be indicated.

The most important work of individual treatment in the case of childhood bereavement is to allow the child a place in which it is safe to experience her feelings and an ally who will be able to help her to do so.

In individual therapy for children, feelings may be expressed through talking or symbolically through play or artwork. In this way, the therapist and the child can understand the child's feelings together.

A therapist will help the bereaved child by facilitating the expression of feelings, then by naming these feelings, and finally by recognizing that these feelings can be talked about, understood, tolerated, and survived.

The therapist's job is to identify the child's feelings when the child cannot name them herself, to accept these feelings as important, and then to clarify their meanings with the child. This process allows the child to think more freely about her own sadness, her own anger, her own feelings of loneliness and abandonment and to struggle actively to figure out how to adapt to life without the person who has been lost. Jacky's story from chapter 3 illustrates this process.

There are a variety of situations that may increase the likelihood that a child will require individual therapy following a loss.

First, if a child's parent is having difficulty supporting her feelings and her mourning because she is overtaxed by the demands being made on her by work, or by financial or emotional stress, the child may need outside help to begin or to continue the mourning process.

Second, if a child returns to earlier ways of acting and if this lasts for more than a few months, this is an indication that the child is not moving forward through her grief and that she might need individual therapy.

Third, if a child is under the age of four or if there are other reasons that she cannot process the loss by herself, then individual therapy may be needed. For example, if the child has particular difficulty relinquishing the conscious or unconscious belief that the loved one continues to exist, therapy is likely to be helpful.

To illustrate, one little girl, referred to in part 1, nineteen-month-old Diane, was told the facts of her other's suicide repeatedly. While she verbally acknowledged them, for the first two weeks after the mother's suicide, she also repeatedly asked about her mother's whereabouts and when she would return.[9]

In the first four weeks of her therapy when she was almost four years old, Diane did not acknowledge her mother's death at all. Only when a game of losing toys was interpreted by the analyst as being like losing the painful feelings that we don't want to feel did Diane show her concern about her mother's death.

For the following ten weeks of therapy, Diane continued to play games where she searched for something that was lost, indicating that she was still looking for her mother and wondering where she had gone.

Because her mother died when she was only a year and a half old and because her therapy took place when she was not even four, Diane did not understand about death. She did not understand that her mother could die and never come back, and she showed her therapist that she still believed that her mother was somewhere, if only she could find her.

Her therapist had to gently remind her over and over again that her mother could not come back. And when she showed how much she wished that she could be with her mother again, the therapist let her know that he understood this wish.

It was through his repeated reminders of the reality of Diane's mother's death and his empathy for her sad wishes to be with her mother again that the therapist was able to help Diane to finally come to the conscious and unconscious acceptance of the fact that her mother no longer existed and then to make a significant attachment to her new stepmother.

Sometimes in therapy a child can also express the anger she cannot express in her outside life. The therapist encourages this, even if the anger is directed at him. One therapist wrote about being called "moose," "dumb," "stupid," and "crazy" by his ten-year-old patient when that child was feeling particularly angry about the death of his father.[10]

In this way, the therapist provided someone safe upon whom the child could turn his aggression.

It is natural that children will feel angry and hurt in response to having been left behind by a loved one who has died. And it is very important for the child to be able to work through these feelings in order to be left with relatively positive feelings toward the person they have lost.

One reason that it is important for a child to have a place to express and understand her anger and aggression is that it is common for children to direct leftover angry feelings toward themselves. As I have mentioned, they may feel that they caused the loved one to leave them because they were not good enough or because they misbehaved. These kinds of feelings can affect the child's self-concept and self-esteem. They may feel bad, no good, and not worthy of love—and these feelings can last a lifetime.

In order to prevent this from happening and to prevent the child from becoming depressed (which is often the result of a child being angry with herself), therapy that allows the expression and understanding of these angry feelings is necessary.

As Drs. Thomas Lopez and Gilbert W. Kliman stated in the case of Diane, "It was the context provided by the analytic relationship as a whole that made mourning possible for Diane."[11]

The individual treatment of a bereaved child or teenager may also serve another function. In the intense contact between the child or teen and the therapist, the child is provided with the opportunity to develop a significant relationship with an understanding and uniquely interested adult.

While it is neither appropriate nor necessary for the therapist or analyst to become a substitute parent, it is often the case that the relationship with the therapist fills a temporary void in the child's or teen's life for a sympathetic ally in the absence of a lost parent or in the case where the parents are not available to help with mourning because they are involved in their own mourning process.

While the relationship between the therapist and the child or teen is designed to help the child or teen to understand her feelings and to work through them, the relationship can also be considered to constitute a considerable support to the child or teen and a relational environment well suited for mourning. Children and teens need continuing love and investment from their parents and other important adults in their lives after a loss. With the loss of one of the parents or of another significant relationship, this need continues and must find an outlet.

Option 5: Cognitive Behavioral Therapy

Cognitive behavioral therapy (CBT) is another form of treatment that may be offered to you or your child. CBT is somewhat different from the individual psychotherapy I have described so far. It is a behavioral therapy that teaches people to change their thinking patterns. A therapist who practices CBT can help the person they work with to change their own thinking in order to cope with difficult situations, evaluate problematic behaviors, and have greater control over their reactions to their emotions.

For example, if a child has experienced a loss, she might have overly negative thoughts about herself based on guilty feelings related to her belief that she contributed to her loss. CBT works on the assumption that once the child becomes aware that her thoughts are incorrect—in this case, that she is not in fact responsible for her loss—she can change her thinking through behavioral strategies.

In a form of therapy called Grief-Help, children are provided with some education about grief and then they are given cognitive behavioral therapy.[12]

In a study done in the Netherlands, this form of help was compared to general supportive therapy for children experiencing prolonged grief disorder (PGD). The children in this study had experienced the death of a loved one and their treatment was combined with parental counseling.

In this study, CBT Grief-Help was made up of several parts. The first part of treatment was titled "Who died?" and invited participants to talk about the circumstances of the loss, what they missed, and what they wished they could still share with the lost person.

This part encouraged the children to confront the reality of the loss and aided therapists in identifying possible maladaptive thinking and behavioral patterns.

The second part of treatment was called "What is grief?" and helped the children make adjustments to bereavement. Bereavement was explained as encompassing four tasks: facing the reality and pain of the loss; regaining confidence in yourself, other people, life, and the future; focusing on your own problems and not on those of others; and continuing activities that you used to enjoy.

During this treatment, participants wrote three letters to an imaginary or real friend to summarize things learned. In this study, Grief-Help provided greater improvements in prolonged grief disorder symptoms as compared to supportive therapy.[13]

Option 6: Family Therapy

In cases where there are a number of family members who are having difficulty following a loss, family therapy may be the best choice. In such a case, it may not be possible for each member of the family to have their own individual therapy due to financial limitations or the difficulty of getting a number of different people in the same family to multiple different appointments. And it may be that the difficulties various family members are having can be addressed together as a family. A death affects all family members and all family relationships, and some families need help adjusting to the changes in the relationships within the family following a loss.

For example, if an older child in the family seems to be taking on the role of family caretaker, this will not only affect that child but it will affect that child's relationships with everyone else in the family. The parent may be sidelined, the siblings may become dependent on the sibling caretaker, and the child who has become the caretaker will be burdened with too much responsibility, whether emotional or actual.

Similarly, if one child is having a great deal of trouble with mourning, this will affect the entire family. That child may get more attention; the other children may become resentful of that child, and the parent or parents may feel overtaxed.

Family therapy can be helpful in all of these situations. It can also be of help when the parent or caregiver needs guidance in modeling their grief, in knowing how allow for emotional expression in the family and in discussing loss with the children.

Here is one description of a family therapy experience. Perihan Rosenthal[14] wrote about a six-year-old girl who was brought to therapy because she had become withdrawn, refused to go to school, complained that she hated her mother, and had threatened suicide, all approximately six months after her father had died by suicide.

In this family, the mother was consumed by her own grief and was having difficulty caring for her three children, who were one, three, and six.

The children were confused about what had happened to their father and whether or not they were responsible for his death.

The therapist decided to see the whole family together rather than just seeing the six-year-old. She helped the mother to talk with her children about what had happened to their father and to explain that their father's suicide was no one's fault.

The therapist also encouraged the mother to talk about the father's problems in simple terms so that the children could better understand why he had taken his life. She suggested that the mother say that their dad had not wanted to live and that although she had asked him to get help for himself, he had refused.

In this way, the mother was able to communicate to the children that their father had serious problems before his death and that she was sure that neither she nor they were responsible for the father's death.

In the course of treatment, the six-year-old began to talk about the fact that she felt her mother was very sad. She explained that she had a theory that this was because her younger sister bothered their mother and made too many demands on her.

Again, the mother, with the help of the therapist, was able to clarify that it was her own grief over her husband's death that made her sad and not any of the behavior of the children.

Additionally, in the course of treatment, the mother was helped to set new limits with the children and to establish a new routine with them, including spending special time with each child individually.

In this case, both the mother and the children were helped by the family treatment. The mother learned how to be more expressive of real circumstances with her children, and she began to understand and address her six-year old's real concerns.

The six-year-old was relieved of her feeling that her sister (and she) were burdens on her mother, and as a result, she improved dramatically in regard to the symptoms she had come in with.

Option 7: Group Therapy

Children who have suffered a loss often find solace in meeting with other children who are in a similar situation—especially shortly after the loss has occurred.

One of the common themes among children and teens who have lost a parent or other loved one is the sense of being alone or of being different from their friends and classmates.

Meeting with other children and teens who have lost a parent can help relieve these feelings of aloneness and can be very supportive.

Groups provide a safe space for children and teens to experience their grief and, when they're ready, to talk about it.

Good groups of this kind allow children and teens to "come as they are," that is, to just be who they are in the group. No demands are made on them, and they are allowed to share their experiences when they choose.

Group activities have all sorts of possibilities, including talking together, doing artwork together, or participating in activities together.

In her study of bereaved children, Jessica Koblenz mentioned a boy who wanted to be a part of such a group but did not know of one. In the absence of one being available, he started a group of his own with three friends who had also lost a parent, which they called "The Dead Parents Club."[15]

So, groups can be formed by children or teens themselves, they can be led by mental health professionals, they can be held at school, or they can be based on a peer counseling model where teens who have experienced a loss help other teens or younger children to deal with their grief.

Option 8: Participation in Programs at a Grief Center

Communities that have a center for grieving children and grieving families are lucky indeed as these centers are rare.

Such centers can provide a variety of services and a much-needed sense of community for families who have lost a loved one.

One such community is Portland, Oregon, where the Dougy Center is located. The Dougy Center offers a wealth of services for children, teens, and adults. They use a peer grief support model for helping children and teens cope before and after the death of a family member.

The Dougy Center model has been replicated in over 500 sites throughout the world. It is considered the gold standard of practice in the field of grief and loss, and they have published numerous pamphlets and booklets that offer specific help and advice (see the Resources section of this book).

Another grief program, and a very innovative one, is located in Bristol, England—but their services are available to people all over the world.

Louis Weinstock, a psychotherapist, started something he calls Apart of Me, a multifaceted program for teens who have experienced loss. It includes an in-app game for mobile devices that teenagers anywhere in the world can play to help them with their grief (see the Resources section for the link).

Apart of Me also offers group experiences for teens to process their grief with peers. Those teens can then learn how to guide others through grief via peer counseling if they like.

In general, groups for children and teens are often organized by age or by type of loss. Some people believe that children and teens who have experienced a loss through suicide benefit most from attending groups with other children and teens who have experienced this type of loss. It is sometimes the case that children and teens who have a close loved one who has died by suicide do not feel they can relate to other forms of loss. And it can also be the case that stories about suicide may be disturbing to children who have lost loved ones in other ways.

Option 9: School-Based Interventions

Public schools in the United States are required to provide help for students who are experiencing difficulties that get in the way of learning.

For this reason, when the loss of a loved one occurs, it is important for the bereaved child's caregiver to contact the child's school as soon as possible in order to inform the school of what has happened and to inquire as to what services are available.

All schools should have a school counselor who can be helpful to the bereaved child, whether by meeting with the child's adult guardians and/or by meeting with the child herself. The school counselor can then relay information to the classroom teachers to help them respond sensitively and appropriately to the child.

Some schools, however, will have more elaborate systems in place to help bereaved children—and the best-prepared schools are those with a multitiered system for dealing with loss among its students.

In such schools there will be at least three levels of intervention. This is the gold standard for dealing with loss—and if your local school does not offer such services, you might ask them to look into developing such a program. Your school can refer to the article written by Jillian Blueford, Nancy Thacker, and Pamelia Bott, the reference for which can be found in the end notes of this book.[16]

In the first level, all students and all personnel will have been provided with ongoing education about loss and how to deal with it. There will be a manual for school staff to refer to in order to help them when a student suffers a loss, and there will be a mechanism for identifying students who are struggling with loss. Safe spaces for bereaved children to go when they need a break from the classroom will have been identified and outfitted in a way that will be comfortable and comforting for children who are grieving.

Level 2 will provide support services to small groups of students experiencing loss and will provide check-ins for each individual student who has suffered a loss.

Level 3 will provide individualized services to children and teens who have experienced a loss, including individual counseling, check-ins, and mentoring.

Children and teens who attend schools with this sort of sophisticated preparation for dealing with loss are, of course, in a great position to get the help they need at school.[17]

In most communities, there are a number of options for helping
grieving children, but in many cases, you must actively seek out these
services. Procuring individual therapy, group therapy, attendance at a
grief center, or even school services will require you to act on behalf of
the grieving child. And this is difficult because often, after a loss, the
adults in the family are overwhelmed with their own grief and with
other responsibilities. The time and energy needed to find a therapist
or other service may be hard to come by—but of course it is important to try to do this.

If you are one such adult, if time, energy, or finances are in short
supply for you, start with exploring what the child's school has to offer
and then check out some of the books and podcasts in the Resources
section of this book.

Here I have described many ways that individual, group, or family
therapy can be helpful for a bereaved child. Having discussed this at
length, I would like to add that deciding to engage a child in therapy,
in a group, or at a grief center must be a thoughtful process which, if
possible, includes the child.

You can talk to your child about what you have noticed about how
they are doing. It is important to do this in a sensitive way. For example, you could say, "I notice you've seemed very sad since Grandma
died and you've spent a lot of your time in your room." Try not to
sound critical or judgmental in any way. At that point you can tell
them what therapy is, what a group is like, what services are available
at their school, or what your local grief center has to offer. Ask if they
think they might like to—or need to—participate in one of these.

They may be interested and they may agree to give it a try, but
there are also times when children will say that they do not want to go
to a group or to therapy or that they are not ready yet. In such cases,
you will have to use your own judgment about what is best. There are

times when a child's feeling of not being ready for therapy or other program can be respected and honored. In such a case, if the child's symptoms are not too severe it may be best to watch and wait for a few weeks or months to see if the child can do better on her own or whether she will come around to accepting the idea of therapy or participation in a group. There are also times when a child's difficulties are so severe that a parent or other family member feels that a child desperately needs help. In this case, the adult should contact their care provider and discuss how to encourage the child to participate in the treatment they need.

Monitoring the Mourning Process

Following a major loss, it is important to monitor how a child or teen is doing.

While the majority of children and teens do well, a significant number have difficulty progressing in their grieving process—or they experience problems with their overall well-being.

It is important for the family to watch how a child is doing and to obtain professional help if there are signs that the mourning process is not moving forward or is going in a direction that is problematic for the child or teen.

So what are some of the signs that a child may need professional help? They might be behaving dramatically differently than they did before they lost a loved one—or they might not be behaving differently or talking about their loss at all. They might seem confused, lost, lonely, depressed, highly anxious, or they might engage in behaviors that are getting them in trouble. If you are noticing these signs several months after the loss, it is likely that their mourning process is not moving along smoothly.

There are a number of possibilities of what might be going wrong, and here I will describe some of the most common of the possibilities. Please note that not all grief professionals use diagnoses, as they feel this pathologizes the grief process; however, it is my belief that having a name for the child's difficulty can be helpful for the caregiver.

Prolonged Grief Disorder or Prolonged Mourning

Prolonged grief disorder (PGD) is the term used by psychiatrists and psychologists to describe grief reactions that are considered to be prolonged or unhealthy.

At times, a child or a teenager may feel very sad and appear to be in mourning for quite a long time. When it seems that they are not able to move through their grief for six months to a year, this is called Prolonged Grief Disorder (PGD) or chronic mourning.

PGD or chronic mourning involves profound feelings of sadness, dejection, loss of self-esteem, and possibly depression. The child or teen might experience unusually intense and prolonged emotional reactions, in many cases with continuing anger and/or anxiety and longing and preoccupation with the lost loved one. The child or teen may also be experiencing any of the following:

- Intense emotional pain
- Guilt
- Denial of the loss
- Blame (toward themselves or someone else)
- Difficulty accepting the death
- Feeling they have lost a part of themselves
- An inability to experience any positive mood
- Emotional numbness
- Difficulty engaging in social or other activities

This diagnosis is given only six or more months after a loss has occurred and includes at least three of the following:

- Disbelief about the death
- Emotional pain regarding the loss
- Difficulty moving on with life
- Emotional numbness
- A sense that life is meaningless
- Intense loneliness nearly every day for at least a month
- Identity disruption
- Avoidance of reminders of the death

For example, Chris was twelve when his father died suddenly. Chris and his father had shared a very good relationship. Chris's father had coached his soccer and Little League teams, and he was athletic and enthusiastic.

When Chris's father died, Chris was extremely upset. He cried for hours after his mother told him the news, and he was very sad for days afterward.

He served as a pallbearer at his father's funeral and was proud to do so.

But as the days went on, Chris became progressively angrier. He complained over and over about how unfair it was that his father had died. He alternated between blaming himself for his father's death, saying that they had practiced too hard the day of the death, and blaming the doctors in the emergency room who were not able to revive his father after his heart attack.

Chris stopped attending soccer and Little League practice. He did not want to play anymore, and instead he spent a great deal of time in his room playing video games.

This went on for several months—and it was clear that Chris just could not accept his father's death nor could he stand any reminders of the activities that he had enjoyed with his father. He was withdrawn, and it was clear that he was very, very lonely.

Chris was stuck in his grief process. He was just not moving through his anger and the devastation he felt about the loss of his father.

Chris's mother was also devastated—but she had enough energy to recognize that her son was in trouble. She took him to see a child psychiatrist, wondering if he needed medication for his anger. The psychiatrist explained that Chris was in mourning, and it was being expressed through his anger. He did not think that medication was the right answer for Chris. He suggested that Chris see a child therapist to work on understanding his feelings about losing his dad, and he gave Chris's mom several names of therapists she could call.

To date, very little is known about exactly what causes PGD in bereaved children and adolescents. But recent research suggests that losing someone, especially a parent, to a chronic illness, losing a mother, feeling one could have done something to prevent the death, a history of depression in the child or teen, and/or a family history of anxiety disorders might put children and teens at risk for PGD. It is known that approximately 3 to 12 percent of parentally bereaved children will develop PGD.[1]

For another example, I met Isaac when he was twenty-seven. Five years out of college, he had an interesting job which fully engaged him. But despite his work and his obvious intelligence, Isaac suffered from a great deal of self-doubt. He was very critical of himself, and he talked frequently about how much better it would have been if he had worked harder in college.

Over the first few sessions, I came to learn that Isaac had a complicated history. His father had died when he was fourteen, and prior to his death his father had suffered from a chronic illness and abused his pain medicine. The father spent most of the last three years of his life in bed, asking various family members to get things for him while simultaneously criticizing them for not doing it well enough.

Isaac came to see me for five years. During this time, he and his wife had two children and he became a very involved father. He rose in the ranks at his job, and his marriage was a good one.

However, Isaac continued to feel critical of himself. He also continued to suffer from a low level of depression and irritability.

As his children started to grow up, I learned more about his unhappiness.

He frequently complained that his mother was not particularly interested in his children and only came to visit when he invited her—and even then, only once or twice a year.

He was very sad that his children did not have a more invested grandmother, and this brought up a great many feelings about his mother and father.

Isaac began to talk about how little he had gotten from his father growing up. There were four children in the family, and his father was not available for any of them. He was frequently out of the house and when he was home, he was harsh and critical of the kids. From the time Isaac was eleven, his father spent most of his time in bed.

Just when Isaac was at the age when he might have been out playing sports and having his father come to his games—or going to sporting or cultural events together—Isaac's father became more unavailable to him than ever as he became more ill.

As the oldest, Isaac frequently argued with his father—and just prior to his father's death, they had one last argument.

It turned out that despite his negative feelings toward his father, Isaac felt badly about this last fight. He also regretted that he had not been able to say goodbye to his father. It was not clear what caused his father's death, but Isaac suspected that his father had taken too many of his pain pills and, whether intentionally or unintentionally, had killed himself. Isaac did not actually blame himself for his father's death—he understood that his father was a troubled man—but he did continue to feel very badly about the way things ended between them.

When his father died, Isaac's mother was quite overwhelmed. She did what she needed to do for the children in terms of preparing meals and getting them to school and doctor appointments, but she provided almost no emotional support.

Three years after his father's death, Isaac's mother started to date a man with whom she became serious very quickly. This man had a child from his previous marriage who was younger than Isaac and his siblings, and the child moved into the home the year that Isaac went to college.

Going forward, Isaac's mother devoted a great deal of energy to her new partner and to his son—and Isaac felt that she did not devote enough energy to him or his siblings. He went through college making his own way and involving himself in a great deal of political activism.

Over time, I came to understand that Isaac's highly ambivalent feelings about his father had made it very hard for him when his father died. Mourning is always complicated when the relationship with the person who died contains intensely mixed feelings.

Isaac had very little support for his mourning process after his father died. He really had no adult to support him—and in fact, he was the main emotional support for his younger siblings.

Isaac internalized his father's criticism of him, and he became very self-critical. He doubted his own abilities and his own work ethic. He was irritable like his father had been, and he was unhappy despite the outward appearance of a successful life.

I came to the conclusion that Isaac suffered from prolonged grief disorder. Because of the complicated nature of his relationship with his father and his almost total lack of support at the time of his father's death and in the years after, he had never really been able to move through a healthy grief process.

Antidepressant medication and continued work in therapy were helpful to Isaac, but his unhappiness and his unresolved grief had lasted a long time and had become a part of him. Fortunately, he was a motivated young man and continued to work hard to understand and work through his complex emotions, especially his sadness around the deprivation he had suffered. However, he did continue to mourn the lack of loving grandparents on his side of the family for his own children.

Incomplete Mourning

A specific form of disordered mourning is called incomplete mourning. This occurs when a child's mourning has begun but has not continued. There are several signs that caregivers can keep an eye out for. Over the course of more than six months, the child might continue to deny that they have experienced a loss by not talking about it or by not expressing sad feelings. They might experience exaggerated and continued aspects of normal grief such as depression, poor appetite, resisting involvement in close relationships, inappropriate identification with the dead parent, too rapid attempts to replace the dead parent, or memorialization of the dead parent.

If any of these are occurring for a prolonged period, it is a good idea for a parent or caregiver to seek out professional help for the child.

For example, Caroline was nineteen when her mother was diagnosed with an inoperable brain tumor. In order to receive this diagnosis, her mother had to endure numerous difficult diagnostic tests, including an angiogram in which dye was injected into her femoral artery and scans were taken of her brain to locate the tumor.

Caroline's mother was treated for six months, to no avail, and she died at home with Caroline and her father at her bedside.

Caroline was initially very sad, but after a month she left for her second year at college where she socialized with her friends and did well academically for the first semester.

Over Christmas vacation, however, Caroline began to experience severe headaches and insisted that she needed to see a neurologist. She was sure that she too had a brain tumor and described symptoms similar to those her mother had experienced. Caroline succeeded in getting the neurologist to order tests including an angiogram, and her belief that she had a tumor continued until the results of the tests and scans came back negative.

What had happened here?

Why had Caroline subjected herself to these extreme medical tests?

Rather than mourning her mother, Caroline had unconsciously become her mother. Rather than feeling sad and alone, she developed the same physical symptoms as her mother had experienced in her last illness.

In other words, Caroline's body took on the mourning that her mind was not able to engage in.

Following Caroline's negative test results, her father insisted that she begin individual psychotherapy. In the course of this therapy, Caroline entered a second period of mourning for her mother during which she experienced the sadness and pain that had been interrupted during her first effort at grief.

Traumatic Shock

Finally, I have come to my own difficulty.

When my father died suddenly, I had a very particular reaction. In order to protect myself from the full impact of my father's death, I froze—physically, emotionally, and psychologically. I remained physically frozen for hours. Psychologically, I remained frozen for years. I did not cry or scream or suffer the dramatic feelings that would be expected following the death of a parent. I coped and carried on and moved through life in an effective but slightly disconnected way.

In the hours after my father died, I sat in a chair in the dining room of my house without thinking or feeling.

This was not something I tried to do. It happened without my knowledge or intention.

When the death of a close loved one—a parent or sibling or friend—happens suddenly or violently or completely unexpectedly, one way of reacting is the way I reacted, with traumatic shock.

Originally a medical term describing the physical reaction to acute injury, I am borrowing this term to apply to acute psychological shock. Also known as acute stress disorder, traumatic shock is the body's response to overwhelming emotions.

Because the mind is unable to fully process or respond to the traumatic event, it freezes, (along with the body) in order to protect the psyche.

Human beings—as well as other forms of life—do not like to be overwhelmed. Our minds and our bodies have developed defense mechanisms to protect us from being overstimulated by too many emotions at once.

One such defense mechanism involved in traumatic shock is dissociation.

This is the "freeze" part of the "fight/flight/freeze" reaction to fear. As we all know, fear can cause some of us to respond with a burst of energy, designed to fight off an enemy. It can cause others of us to run, to get away from what is threatening us. And still others will freeze, as I did, like a possum that has been cornered.

In humans, this freeze response is also called dissociation. Extremely traumatic events can sometimes cause a person to psychologically disconnect from either themselves or the people around them—or both.

People who experience this may feel disconnected from reality and from their own thoughts and their own feelings, just as I did. This can happen in the case of a sudden death, or during or after any of a multitude of other very frightening events.

Not infrequently, this dissociation will last for quite a while in a lesser form—as it did for me. In this case, people who have experienced a terrible event will not fully process what has happened for a very long time. There may be gaps in their memory of the event, or they may see it again and again in their imaginations just as if it were a video recording.

And freezing—or dissociating—is something we do because the events assaulting us are unbearable.

In the moment, we unconsciously hit the pause button so that we do not have to entirely face what we cannot tolerate facing.

As Natasha Trethewey wrote about her mother's death (which occurred when she was nineteen) in her memoir, *Memorial Drive,* "The whole time I have been working to tell this story, I have done so incrementally, parsing it so that I could bear it: neat, compartmentalized segments that have allowed me to carry on these many years."[2]

In the case of traumatic shock, it may be a long while before the child or teen is ready to unpack their feelings about what has happened. If a parent notices that their child or teen seems dissociated—distant and disconnected—after a loss, they can try to talk with the child about how they are doing. They can gently try to explore how frightening the loss was for the child, and they can try to engage the child in psychotherapy with a therapist who is able to approach the treatment slowly. And the reason that I use the words "gently" and "slowly" is that a person who has dissociated has done so for a good reason. They know instinctively that they are not ready or able to face the reality of what has happened. And, as a result, their defenses against recognizing their painful reality must be respected and only gradually confronted—whether by a parent or a therapist.

Traumatic Bereavement

Traumatic bereavement occurs when a loss is suffered as the result of terrible circumstances such as a mass shooting, suicide, murder, natural disaster, or the like or when a particular loss is especially difficult and overwhelming for a child.

But before looking further at traumatic bereavement let's define the word *trauma*.

These days this term is used all the time. But it really should not be. Trauma is not just anything that happens that it is hard. It is actually an event that is truly overwhelming to an individual—and what is overwhelming for one person may not be overwhelming for another.

So, for example, the loss of a parent for a child who only has one parent may be especially traumatizing and overwhelming for that child. They may be truly traumatized—while the loss of a parent for a child whose parents are divorced and who rarely saw the parent who died may not be traumatizing. While it might be difficult and sad, it may not feel extremely overwhelming.

Bessel van der Kolk, an expert on trauma, defines it this way: "Trauma is specifically an event that overwhelms the central nervous system [of an individual], altering the way [they] process and recall memories." He says that "Trauma is not the story of something that happened back then but, rather, . . . It is the current imprint of that pain, horror, and fear living inside people now."[3]

Vivien Dent, an expert on trauma, has added an important point.[4] She notes that in order for a child to be deeply traumatized, in addition to the traumatizing event there is also usually an absence of adequate soothing and containment following the event. What she means by this is that following trauma, there is usually such chaos that the comfort and reassurance the child needs to recover well is often unavailable—and this is part of what leads to the child being truly traumatized.

In other words, whether a child experiences an event as traumatic will be determined in part by the availability of close loved ones immediately following the event, the child's ability to take in soothing and reassurance from their loved ones, and the child's attachment history and attachment style prior to the trauma.

The experience of trauma is also defined by several other factors:

- The magnitude of the threat experienced (the greater the threat, the more likely it is that it will provoke a trauma response)
- The person's developmental level at the time of the event (with younger children and people who are at a lower developmental level being more likely to be traumatized)
- The person's temperament
- The person's history of previous trauma (with people who have experienced previous trauma being more likely to be retraumatized)
- The meaning the event has for the person following the event[5]

Children and teens may also be traumatized vicariously—that is, they may be traumatized by being with a parent or friend who has experienced an event as traumatizing and who is incapable of reflecting on the event sufficiently to process it.

The results of traumatization are severe. Without help, and without others with whom to share and process their feelings, children may experience a change in their attitude toward life and a sense that things can never be the same again, which may predispose them to a notion of limited future possibility.[6] They may also continue to be anxious, they may continue to be depressed, they may suffer from nightmares and flashbacks and vulnerability to further traumatization for the rest of their lives.

So, now that we have a better idea of what trauma is, we can talk about traumatic bereavement.

Children who lost a parent on 9/11 in the attack on the World Trade Center or who lost a first-responder parent often felt overwhelmed by the enormity of their loss and the circumstances surrounding it. Many were not at home when they found out about the attacks, and many suffered great anxiety about their parents before finding out that one or both had died.

Many of these children required an enormous amount of help in the years following 9/11, and they would be examples of children who were traumatically bereaved.

Children who lose a parent during wartime in their own countries or whose homes or schools are beset by violence, natural disasters, or mass shootings, who do not receive a great deal of soothing and support immediately after the event, and whose ability to respond adaptively is compromised can also be said to have been traumatically bereaved.

Some children and teens who were at the scene of a mass shooting can be said to be traumatically bereaved even if they did not know any of the people who were shot, while others at the same scene may be horrified but not actually traumatized.

In a study on the effect of mass shootings on teenagers, it was found that the majority of young people recover from this sort of trauma and their functioning will return to levels similar to what they were prior to the event within a few months. Meanwhile, a smaller proportion of those children or teens exposed to this kind of event will experience chronic and severe dysfunction. In these cases, treatment by an experienced professional is necessary.[7]

The indirect effects of school shootings are also important to mention here. Children brought up in the last several decades have often experienced a kind of culture of fear within their schools. They experience frequent lockdown drills or actual lockdown events, and this may also be traumatizing to sensitive or especially vulnerable children in and of itself without their having witnessed any actual violence. These children are not traumatically bereaved—but they may be traumatized.

PTSD Related to Bereavement

Posttraumatic stress disorder (PTSD) is one of the many possible outcomes of traumatic bereavement.

PTSD is a diagnosis which has been around for decades, and, like "trauma," it is a term used casually by many people when they are describing how they feel after a particularly difficult event. But in clinical terms, actual PTSD involves more than this. A child or teen who has PTSD will be experiencing intense, disturbing thoughts and feelings related to the traumatic event they have experienced. These feelings last long after the traumatic event has ended. These children may relive the event through flashbacks or nightmares. They may frequently feel sadness, fear, or anger, and they may feel detached or estranged from other people. Children with PTSD may avoid situations or people that remind them of the traumatic event, and they may have strong negative reactions to something as ordinary as a loud noise or an accidental touch.

A diagnosis of PTSD requires that the child have experienced or witnessed a disturbing event, or they have learned that a traumatic event has happened to a close family member or friend. It can also occur as a result of repeated exposure to horrible details of trauma.[8]

PTSD related to bereavement is a bit different. It involves the usual symptoms of posttraumatic stress disorder but occurs only after a loss. It features intrusive thoughts that revolve around the death event itself, leading individuals to avoid internal and external reminders of the event.[9]

The professional literature suggests that there are certain factors that make it more likely that a child or teen will develop PTSD. Some of these include being female, being younger (ages two to nine), and belonging to a lower socioeconomic status.

Young children aged two to nine have increased rates of PTSD when exposed to direct or indirect violence. Older children and teens may need multiple exposures to violence for it to lead to PTSD, suggesting that younger children are more sensitive to violence and more likely to develop psychological symptoms after being exposed to violence.

For example, Tina was eight when her parents had a violent argument in the parking lot of her younger brother's daycare center. This argument was one of many her parents had had over the prior year. But what made this particular morning different is that Tina's father had bought a handgun recently and had brought it with him when he came to the daycare parking lot. As the argument escalated, Tina's father shot his wife and then himself.

This horrific event affected Tina and her brother in a multitude of ways. Tina's brother was only three years old at the time, and though he was inside his daycare during the argument and saw nothing, he did hear the bang of the gun. From that day on, he was easily startled by loud noises and often cried inconsolably when surprised. He missed his mother desperately and struggled between missing his father and feeling terribly angry with him.

Tina was not at the daycare at the time of the shooting, but she was old enough to understand exactly what had happened after she was told. Her aunt tried to be gentle as she spoke to her, but Tina immediately became anxious and frightened. From that moment on, Tina shied away from her male relatives, she was frightened by loud noises or sudden movements, and she refused to go anywhere near her brother's old daycare when going out in the car. In fact, she would not ride in the car at all until whomever was driving promised her that they would not go down the street where the daycare was located. At night she had nightmares and could not be comforted when she woke up from them. For the first few months after her parents' deaths, she was withdrawn. She did not want to engage with friends or with her aunt and uncle with whom she now lived.

Tina had a terrible case of bereavement-related PTSD. She needed years of help of all kinds, including therapy targeted at loss and PTSD. And her therapy was not easy. She rejected several of the first therapists who tried to be of help to her. Finally, when she was around sixteen she settled on one therapist with whom she felt she could talk. But even this therapy was difficult. Tina struggled with ambivalent feelings toward her therapist. It was hard for her to trust anyone and this was demonstrated through her feelings about her therapist. After a couple of years she slowly began to process some of her feelings about her parents, their deaths, and her resulting difficulties with closeness with the people in her life.

If you have a child in your life who has experienced a traumatic bereavement, remember that processing their experience will be a difficult journey and it is likely that it will take them years to do so.

Also:

- They will need a great deal of reassurance and soothing immediately after the event and for the weeks, months, and possibly years, following the event.
- Going forward, it will be important to distinguish between what happened at the time of the event and what is happening in the here and now. Traumatized people often confuse

the two. A good saying for them is "That was then. This is now."

- After a traumatic bereavement, the child or teen will require individual psychotherapy, and the parents should also attend occasional sessions with the child's therapist to better understand how to help their child or teen.

Absence of Mourning

Absence of mourning is a stark contrast to loss-related PTSD.

We call it an absence of mourning when children show few or no signs of mourning at all for six months or more after a loved one has died.

While it is quite normal for children to be in a state of shock following the death of a much-loved friend or relative, this state generally only lasts for a few days or weeks.

And while some children are unable or unwilling to talk about what has happened or what they feel, and while they may want to go on with planned activities, this can be considered normal if it only goes on for a few weeks or months. It is worrisome if they continue to do this for more than six months.

Danny was eleven when his father died. When he was thirteen, his mother called me to schedule an appointment. She was very worried about the fact that Danny had never cried about his father's death and had spoken very little about his father since his death.

When I evaluated Danny I had the difficult task of determining whether his lack of reaction to his father's death was a developmentally appropriate and expectable response or whether he was suffering from an absence of mourning.

After a few sessions, Danny started to talk a little about his father. He said that he did miss his father, but that he found it very hard to talk to anyone about it. He felt that talking to his mother would just make her sadder than she already was, and he did not feel his friends would understand if he talked to them. He was also afraid of crying in front of his friends, which is what he thought might happen if he brought up the subject of his father's death.

Danny was on the cusp of adolescence, an awkward time when children often feel especially self-conscious. It was difficult for Danny to know how to talk about his sadness and whom to talk to about it. However, he was not experiencing an absence of mourning. He did feel sad about his father's death and he could talk about this with me. He was thinking about his father and what it meant to no longer have his father in his life.

I thought that the thing that would be most helpful for Danny would be to have a group of other kids to talk with who had also experienced loss. When I found such a group and recommended that he go, Danny was willing. And although quiet in the group, Danny did participate occasionally, and he told his mother that it was good to know that he was not the only one who had the experience of losing a parent.

Similarly, it is possible to misidentify an absence of mourning in younger children. Small children may sometimes look like they are not sad or mourning because they are so involved in playing, even right after a loss. When children under the age of six experience a death, they can often be seen to play and socialize as if nothing has happened. But this is different from an absence of mourning.

Often children will play and enjoy times with friends in between periods of sadness. And if you watch their play closely you may even see evidence that they are playing out some parts of what has happened with their loss.

Often it takes time for a young child to understand and to accept that a loved one has actually died and is never coming back. So true mourning may not develop for several weeks or months. Frequently the young child's grief reaction is expressed indirectly or in symbolic form—in their play, in their artwork, in difficulties with sleep or eating, or in crankiness or upset about other things.

Delayed Mourning

Sometimes a child does not start mourning until quite a while after their loss. We call this delayed mourning when it starts more than six months after the death.

Patricia was twelve when her father died in a motorcycle accident. She accepted his death and went on with her life without showing many sad feelings. She did well in school, had fun with her friends, and helped her mother with her two younger brothers.

This continued for two years, until Patricia was fourteen. Then one day her mother was called by the school to say that Patricia was in the nurse's office crying uncontrollably. When her mother came to pick her up, Patricia could not explain what she was feeling.

When Patricia came in to see me, she looked sad and downtrodden. She told me that she didn't know what was wrong with her.

When I asked her more about herself, Patricia told me that she had recently moved from the house where they had lived when her father was still alive. She couldn't say much more so I asked if she could draw a picture of the house.

She drew what she called a "rainbow heart" over a tiny house. The picture was of a many-colored heart with a large crack down the middle.

I asked if perhaps Patricia was very sad because she and her family had moved away from the place where she was last able to be with her father and if perhaps the heart that was breaking was hers.

She nodded yes.

This drawing and Patricia's acknowledgement of its meaning allowed me to start to understand her sadness and to talk about all the ways she had kept these feelings inside for so long in order to be a "good girl."

Mourning can be delayed by a child either for a short time or for a very long time. It is often not obvious that this is occurring as the child may seem to be coping well and continuing on with her life.

Often the adults around the child are pleased at how well the child is doing.

However, when a child does not mourn the loss of a significant relationship, there is a toll to be paid. Like Patricia, children may function well, presumably in order to maintain self-esteem and to avoid painful feelings, but this good level of functioning can be quite superficial.

Deep feelings and the work of mourning may be kept away and may only emerge when there is a trigger that stirs them up and brings them to the surface.

Sometimes a child will not cry or seem sad after a loss. If this lasts for a few days—or even a few weeks or a couple of months—this can be part of a normal mourning process. But if, over time, the child does not seem sad, does not want to talk about the lost loved one, and does not show signs at home or at school that she is processing the loss, it will be important to get some professional help to aid the child in beginning to acknowledge and work through her grief.

Similarly, if a child who did not seem particularly sad initially suddenly becomes sad or depressed a year or more after a loss, this may also be a sign of delayed grief

Maturational Grief

Grief researchers Patricia Johnson and Paul Rosenblatt described something they called maturational grief. They said that following the loss of a parent, a child may reexperience grief at a variety of points in the process of growing up. They found that in most cases, this is actually quite common and not in any way a sign of pathological grief.

They said that at each new developmental stage, the child needs to reprocess their grief and to understand it at a higher level—and this often involves feeling the sad feelings all over again. This is actually necessary for the child so that as they grow they can understand their loss in a way that is in keeping with their new level of maturity.[10]

For example, Mari was eight when she lost her father. At twenty-four she came to see me for psychotherapy. She was a smart, beautiful, sensitive young woman, but she was very sad.

She had just entered a Ph.D. program, and she was aware that she was missing her father. We talked about how strange this was for her since it had been so long since her father had died. But she was an extremely insightful person, and she quickly realized how powerfully she wished he had been able to see her at this point in her life. She thought he would have been proud that she was going for her Ph.D., and she wished she could talk with him about her courses and about her research.

Mari remembered her father as a kind and empathic man, and she felt that she could use his support at this point. She had moved to a new city to attend graduate school and felt quite alone.

I urged her to talk with her older siblings and her mother about her father. And when she did, she started to realize that perhaps she had idealized him a bit in her memory. Her mother had loved her father very much, but she told Mari that her father could be self-absorbed at times and that he had been very involved in his own work as a lawyer. He worked long hours and was often not home for the first fifteen years of their marriage.

Mari was the youngest of three, and she had been born at the point in his career when her father was successful enough that he did not have to work as many hours. As a result, she got more of his attention than her two siblings or even his wife had.

By talking more deeply with her mother and siblings and by understanding other perspectives regarding her father, Mari was able to revise some of her idealization of him, to deepen her relationship with some of the members of her nuclear family, and to remember and re-mourn her father at a new developmental stage in her life.

She only came to see me for about six months because her difficulties were not particularly entrenched. She was very sad that she had lost her father so early in her life, she was sad that her father had missed so much of her life, and she had needed to give herself the opportunity to mourn the loss of his seeing her as a Ph.D. candidate. And then she was ready to move forward, having unburdened herself of the most painful of these feelings.

Re-mourning years after a loss does not necessarily indicate the presence of incomplete mourning. While incomplete grief may need in-depth therapeutic intervention, grief experienced as a result of maturation typically needs only supportive reassurance that such grief is normal and that it occurs frequently for those who have lost a significant person early in life. And, sometimes, a child, teen, or adult may come to therapy with symptoms they do not understand and it may turn out that their symptoms are caused by sadness and maturational grief they were unaware of.[11]

Maturational grief is commonly seen, for example, when bereaved children experience a birthday or graduation. Although the death of the parent may have occurred years in the past, the child feels sad on the day of the event. If consciously experienced, the child recognizes anew that the parent is not there to celebrate and may feel sad, even though the actual event is a happy one.

When not consciously experienced, the child may need help from a supportive adult to realize that they are sad because their beloved parent is not present on their big day.

Katherine was thirteen when her father died of a massive heart attack. She was intensely sad for months following his death but recovered gradually and resumed life as an outgoing, academically talented teen. When it came time to graduate from high school she looked forward to her graduation and to all the festivities surrounding it.

On the actual day of graduation, however, she found that she was not hungry for breakfast, and she felt down in the dumps. When her mother asked what was going on, Katherine replied that she had no idea, she just didn't feel great.

Katherine's mother was well aware of the absence in their life. She herself was missing her late husband and wishing that he could be there to see their daughter graduate. She asked Katherine gently if maybe she might be thinking about all the pictures that would be taken at graduation and the fact that her father would not be in any of them.

Katherine cried for a few minutes and admitted that this was really sad for her.

And then she asked her mother to make pancakes.

High school graduation was one of many milestones that Katherine's father did not live to see, and as each of these milestones occurred, Katherine mourned her father's death again.

*   *   *

There are a variety of pathological variations on the grief process. Here I have mentioned several of these. It is important to recognize the signs and symptoms of each so that you can obtain help for your child or family member should they need it.

CHAPTER 11

Long-Term Support

Following a loss there will be months and years of grief, mourning, and learning to live with loss.

The child who has lost a close loved one will have numerous opportunities to remember the person she has lost and to miss them.

She will have countless moments of loneliness and sadness.

She may have many dreams and nightmares about the person she has lost.

And she will have plenty of thoughts and feelings.

As each new year comes along and she matures, she will re-mourn her loss at a new level.

Each time there is a parents' day or a grandparents' day at school, she will mourn again.

Each Mother's Day or Father's Day, she will feel her loss.

But she will also begin to forget certain things about the loved one she has lost—and this may be upsetting. A gradual process of forgetting is natural but worrisome for the child or teen who only has a few memories to hang on to.

In this section, I will discuss more of the ways that families, friends, and teachers can help bereaved children and teens. I will talk about the process of gradual forgetting, the myth that there is "closure" after a significant loss, and the additional or secondary losses that accompany a death. I will also talk about the surprising fact that positive growth can be experienced from the experience of loss.

* * *

Nothing can remove the pain of loss for a child or teenager who loses a parent or a very close loved one like a sibling or a best friend, but some things *can* be done to help the child as they navigate the new terrain of loss.

First of all, a child who has lost a loved one will often feel starved for attention. Anything that they received from the parent, sibling, or friend who died is now unavailable. And they may feel that there is no hope for retrieving that attention in the future.

Whether you are a parent or a friend or close relative, you can acknowledge the child's fear and you can also try to provide extra attention and support.

This is particularly important because children and teens who have lost a parent or a close loved one may withdraw socially. They may feel different, and they may worry about being perceived as different by other kids. They may feel unsure how to be and what to say to new people. It is especially hard for a child to be sociable when she feels different and sad.

Parents and other close relatives and friends can encourage the bereaved child to start new activities or to go on play dates. They can find ways to make doing this easier for the child, such as accompanying them.

Teachers can make a point of helping the bereaved child or teen join a group at recess or at lunch, and they can continue to monitor how the child is doing socially.

Many of the changes that occur in a child's life as a result of the loss they have suffered cannot be prevented. In this case, sensitivity on the part of all the child's caretakers and school personnel to the added difficulties that these changes pose for the child will be extremely important.

Losses like these are called secondary losses, and they can occur at any time after an initial loss.

Secondary Losses

Secondary losses accompany a greater loss. They are the losses contained within the experience of the loss of a parent or other close loved one. And these losses can also feel like major losses for a child.

These losses include things like having less money or having to move to a new house or apartment, having to change schools, or having a parent who was previously at home have to go to work all day.

These changes can take months—or longer—to adapt to. The child may feel lonely and displaced for quite a while.

When a child's parent becomes ill or dies, when parents divorce, or a parent who was a major wage earner loses their job, the family may have to make a variety of changes to their lifestyle.

If the family moves, the child may have to leave friends and transfer to a different school. School is often an enormous part of a child's world and leaving one school to start at a new one is a huge change for a child and involves many losses within it—including the loss of best friends and familiar classmates, the loss of the well-known school building and neighborhood, the loss of teachers and coaches and others the child has known over time.

Being aware of how difficult this is for a child or teen is the first step you can take to be helpful—but beyond this, it may be possible to help the child further. Talking with the child or teen about what it is like for them is crucial, as is trying to help them to make some initial contacts in the new neighborhood and at the new school.

For example, DJ was seven when his father died. Because his father was the main income earner in his family, DJ and his mother and three brothers had to move in with his mother's parents when they could no longer afford their apartment. The family also no longer had enough money for birthday parties or new clothes.

DJ lost more than his father. He lost his home, his neighborhood, his school, his friends, his daily routine, and his whole way of life. He had to get used to living with his grandparents (who were very strict) as well as getting used to a new school and new kids.

What a child experiences when a loved one dies or leaves depends on so many things: the family's financial circumstances, the amount of community support they have or do not have, and the emotional stability of the remaining family members. These factors—and others—will all affect the child's experience of loss.

The impact of other losses that accompany the initial loss cannot be underestimated. The loss of home or school or neighborhood can be enormous for a child and can have many reverberations throughout her life, both current and future. She may be very sad about the loss of her loved one and also very sad about the fact that she had to move and leave her friends behind. Having multiple losses at one time intensifies the complexity and the depth of grief and mourning for a child or teenager.

Dreams, Nightmares, and Imagined Presences

Immediately after a loss—or for many months or years following a loss—children and teens may have dreams or nightmares where they see the person who has died. Or they may feel that they have seen the ghost of the person or felt their presence. This is quite normal—and in fact, many adults have the same experiences. The wish to be with the lost loved one is powerful and comes out in many ways, including in dreams and imagined presences.

I had frequent dreams about my father after his death. I often dreamed that I saw him in a restaurant or found him hiding in a closet. In each of these dreams I would feel great relief, saying to myself, "I knew it! I always knew he wasn't really dead!" But then, waking up, I would feel disappointed and sad all over again, knowing that this had just been a dream.

The desire to deny a painful reality lives in all of us. In my dreams I could find my father and I could realize a hoped-for event: he hadn't really died! But waking up reminded me that there was a big difference between what I wished for and what was real.

If a child or teen reports having had such a dream, talk about it with them. Ask them what they felt in the dream, and how it felt to wake up from it. Ask them what they think the dream means. If they are having trouble talking about it, you can tell them (using the example of my own dream) that you think that the dream is an indication of how much they miss their loved one and how much they wish the loved one were still alive.

Dreams are a way that we deal with painful feelings and difficult problems we have not been successful at solving during the day. Educating your child or teen about the purpose of dreams and getting them interested in remembering and thinking about their dreams can be quite helpful in aiding them to reflect on their own feelings and their own internal processes.

Gradual Forgetting

One thing that is especially difficult about losing a loved one is that over time, the memories of that person fade. Time spent with them, their appearance, their voice, their mannerisms may all disappear from memory.

Séamas O'Reilly, whose mother died when he was five, writes, "I first realized I'd erased my mother when I was eight. It was Mother's Day . . . I wrote down ten . . . clear memories. My internal accounting had fooled me into thinking my stock was larger than it was."

He says that over time the number of memories he had of his mother became fewer and fewer. He felt bereft when he recognized this. And after several years, he realized that he only had five clear memories of her. He had not written down the original ten, and five of them were gone.

As a boy, O'Reilly realized with surprise how little he remembered his mother. As an older teen, looking back on his mother's death, O'Reilly felt even more pain at realizing he did not remember even as much as he had a few years earlier.

He describes not just the sadness of forgetting, but also the shame he felt. He says that losing so many of his memories of his mother made him think of himself as a "bad and unfeeling son." He describes feeling great remorse, not realizing that the forgetting was beyond his control.[1]

Natasha Trethewey describes a similar experience: "Five years after my mother was gone . . . It had been long enough that the first things I would come to lose of her had already begun to dissipate—what she smelled like, how she walked—and I felt that I was enacting a kind of betrayal, letting her go in pieces."[2]

We imagine that we will always remember certain moments and certain people in our lives; we plan special trips and festive occasions in order to "make memories." But memory is complicated and idiosyncratic. We do not control what we remember and what we forget. And when someone we love dies, we feel disloyal if we do not remember as much as we think we should about them.

Children who experience loss are particularly vulnerable. Even those who lose loved ones as teenagers may find that they remember alarmingly little about the person. And those who lose loved ones before they reach adolescence may remember very little indeed.

At this point in my own life, I have very few memories of my father. I can see him sitting at the head of the dining room table, cutting a piece of fruit; I can visualize him at breakfast, eating a slice of melon, I remember going out to dinner with him at restaurants, and I remember a few times he took care of injuries I had. But considering that he was in my life for fourteen years, I remember surprisingly little.

One thing that may happen for children and teens in the event of a significant loss is that they may begin to cling to objects that link them to their lost loved. And these objects may become more and more valuable as memories fade.

As O'Reilly says, "Lacking the memories to form a coherent sense of [my mother] in my head, I relied instead on what I could see of her around me. . . . She was the giant, lovely photograph in the good room, and the smiling face in a few other family portraits throughout the house. She was the printed-out brochures for her anniversary masses, and the small, laminated mass cards that were placed in a few of the bedrooms."[3]

Often children, adolescents, and even adults find ways to retrieve and create memories. O'Reilly says, "As I got older, I realized there were other people's memories that could fill the gaps, and having heard all the tales of how wonderful she was—and she really was—I found that I delighted more in hearing the scant few negative stories I could wring out of those who knew Mammy best."[4]

As Séamas O'Reilly says, the collective memory can sometimes stand in for the personal. The stories of friends and family can be comforting and can pad the dwindling memory of the child.

O'Reilly describes his pleasure in this: "Telling old stories is a large percentage of what we do when we return home. We sit around the huge kitchen table . . . around that table no one finishes a sentence, and we delight in each other's misremembered notions, undigested memories, embarrassing acts from the past—recollections of Mammy, of each other, of ourselves."[5]

The Myth of Closure

Some people believe that after a death, there are ways to achieve what they call "closure." And by this they mean that there are ways to say goodbye to someone after they die that can allow the loved ones to put that loss in the past.

After my father's death I found myself confused by this idea. I knew that there was no way that his death would stop affecting me. There was no way that I would ever completely get over having lost him as a young teenager, and I knew that there was absolutely no way that I would stop thinking about him.

But every day we hear people talking about their need for closure.

When someone has died or when there has been another sort of loss, people often complain that without closure, they cannot move on.

Sigmund Freud first wrote about mourning in his paper, "Mourning and Melancholia." In it, he talked about the need on the part of the bereaved person to go through each of his memories about the lost loved one and to recognize, each time, that the loved one no longer exists. In this way, Freud said, the mourner can gradually remove the energy he invested in the loved one.

Freud thought that the removal of this energy from the internal relationship with the loved one was necessary. He said that it is only when this process has been completed that the mourner can invest his love in a new person.[6]

But I did not stop investing in the relationship with my father after he died. He was the only father I had ever had and the only father I would ever have. It was clear to me that my relationship with him would continue to be important to me throughout my life. I knew I would continue, over the years, to try to bring my father to mind, to remember who he had been and what effect he had had on me. I knew I would be sad, and I knew that I would continue to feel both relieved and tremendously cheated that he had died when he did. I did not consider the possibility that closure would be forthcoming, nor did I think I needed it.

It is true that I withdrew some of the energy I had previously invested in my relationship with my father. After all, he was no longer there to interact with, nor could I depend on him or his love anymore. But I certainly continued to invest a significant amount of energy in my internal relationship with him.

Pauline Boss has studied this matter, and it turns out that, had I talked to her as a teenager, she would have agreed with me. She calls the idea that closure is necessary "the myth of closure."

She says, "Continuing to use the term 'closure' perpetuates the myth that losses and grief have a prescribed time for ending . . . and that it's emotionally healthier to close the door on suffering than to face it and learn to live with it."[7]

Anyone who has lost a loved one in childhood—or at any time in life—knows that sadness continues, remembering continues, and suffering continues.

When I was a teenager at college, I stood outside looking at the night sky thinking about my father. And often, I spoke to him. He had died when I was fourteen and when I went to college, alone in a new place, having to make new adaptations of all sorts, I missed him all over again. I had not experienced closure at his funeral or in the three years following his death. His absence was always with me, especially in new circumstances. When I felt alone, I needed to call on him to feel a sense of not being *so* alone.

He had died, but he was still with me—as a memory but also as a part of myself. I could imagine his voice and even what he might say to me—and this was both comforting and guiding.

Pauline Boss goes on to say that after suffering, it is important to acknowledge our losses, to name them, find meaning in them, and let go of the quest for closure.

And this is true for children and teens as well.

But children—and even teenagers—are also different from adults. They need the help of those around them to do as Boss says—to name their feelings, to acknowledge these feelings, to find meaning in their loss, and to avoid the temptation to shut down or ignore the pain.

So, who is right—Pauline Boss or the famous Sigmund Freud?

Well, perhaps the truth is somewhere in the middle.

For a person of any age to move forward in the mourning process, some of the energy they invested in the lost loved one *does* need to be freed up so that energy is available to invest in new people and new relationships.

And it may be that, as in the case of a soldier missing in action, when the body has not been found or the cause of the death has not been identified, it is far more difficult for the mourners to remove energy from the loved one and from the circumstances in which they died because there are still so many questions about what happened and why.

It is clear that seeking complete closure may be impossible and the effort can come at a cost. Boss says that too avid a search for closure, too much energy being put into bringing our mourning to an end, can sap us and distract us from other coping options that might lead to growth. If we look and hope for closure, we may resist seeing and valuing the parts of ourselves that have been influenced by the lost loved one. We may miss the resilience that comes from living with the ambiguity of having lost someone dear while still being able to move forward in life.

In Boss's view, closure cuts off the real and symbolic connections to those we have left behind.

For children, I believe, these enduring connections enrich the child's personality and emotional repertoire. The child who remembers his grandpa's sense of humor tries to be funny himself. The teenager who learned from her mother how to love and care for her younger siblings, continues to be empathic and helpful to these siblings after her mother's death. For such a child or teen, the memory of the lost loved one becomes more than a memory—it becomes part of who they are as people.

So, perhaps mourning can occur in an acute way—both for children and adults—it can go on for weeks and months, or even for a couple of years, and then it can simmer down into something that can be lived with. We can miss our loved ones, we can remember them, we can identify with some of their characteristics and internalize these so that we carry part of them with us, and we can be sad from time to time when we especially miss them. And we can do this while we also move forward in our lives.

Neither we adults nor the children we care for need to close our mourning off from our day-to-day life. We do not need complete closure. Mainly, we need to move through the most painful days and weeks of sadness and missing feelings and into a life where we allow ourselves to feel what we feel while we also live normal lives.

As Boss says, instead of searching for closure, we need to look for meaning and new hope.

Growth from Loss

Many people, including children and teens, not only manage to survive difficult losses, but they can grow as the result of their experience with loss.

Scientists who study trauma and loss have found a variety of positive psychological changes following challenging life experiences.

Lawrence Calhoun and Richard Tedeschi called this "posttraumatic growth." They mentioned the following positive changes as being prominent for many people:

- Greater appreciation of life
- Greater appreciation and strengthening of close relationships
- Increased compassion and altruism
- The identification of new possibilities or a purpose in life
- Greater awareness and utilization of personal strengths
- Enhanced spiritual development
- Creative growth

And, as it turns out, one crucial factor that allows people to turn a difficult event into one that promotes growth is the extent to which they explore their thoughts and feelings around that event.

Being willing to admit that a difficult event has occurred appears to be the first step in growing from the experience. As we know, many people prefer to avoid thinking about the bad things that happen to them, and they push away painful feelings about these events.

However, Calhoun and Tedeschi found that the ability to acknowledge that the event has happened and to think about and process the painful feelings associated with the event is what allows some people to grow from their difficult experiences.[8]

Two more researchers, Todd Kashdan and Jennifer Kane, also studied this subject. Using a group of college students, they looked at how much people tended to avoid difficult and painful thoughts and feelings versus how much they were willing to allow them. In their study, the most frequently reported traumas included the sudden death of a loved one, motor vehicle accidents, witnessing violence in the home, and natural disasters.

Kashdan and Kane found that the greater the distress was, the greater the posttraumatic growth that resulted from it—but only in those people who did not avoid their feelings, or who did so infrequently.

Those people who reported greater distress and who did not avoid their feelings reported experiencing the highest levels of growth and meaning in life compared to people who tended to avoid their feelings more.[9]

These findings support the benefits of encouraging children to experience and talk about their feelings following loss. It also supports the importance of having children and teens who are having difficulty experiencing or expressing their feelings get involved in some form of expressive psychotherapy, whether that be individual, group, or family therapy—or even encouraging them to play the grief-oriented video game I referred to earlier created by Apart of Me (see Resources for the link.).

Jessica Koblenz specifically studied children who had lost a parent to find out what helps and what hinders them in their grief process. She also found that there is growth from loss. One child in her study said they had a heightened sense of life and didn't want to waste time or have regrets. Another said he had become more independent. Some mentioned that they learned to seek help from those who were able to provide it. Some found that exercise was a good method for coping with painful feelings, and others found humor helpful.

Teigan, the young woman I met through Winston's Wish who I referred to earlier, told me that what happened to her after she lost her mother shaped what she wanted to do with her life. She described how one of her teachers at school called her every week after her mother died and provided her with much needed attention, support, and guidance. This teacher was an inspiration for Teigan, and she had decided to become a grief counselor for children and teens so that she could help other students, just as her teacher had helped her. In the meantime, she was training to lead grief groups just like the one she had participated in herself.

In the end, Koblenz said that the participants in her study found that loss gets easier as you get older but that grieving is a lifelong process.[10]

And, as Louis Weinstock, founder of Apart of Me, said at a recent conference, "Grief can be a gateway to greater meaning and greater purpose in life."

CONCLUSION

For a child, losing a loved one is scary—because it makes death real.

For a child, death itself is scary—because what *is* death, anyway?

For a child, losing a loved one is excruciating—because the pain of not having the loved one is so terrible and the capacity for bearing pain is so small.

For a child, missing the loved one is possibly the hugest part of loss.

For a child, losing a loved one is confusing—because it is hard to understand why this person had to die.

For a child, losing a loved one stirs up guilt—because the child imagines that she could have prevented her loved one from dying if only she had behaved differently.

And for each child, grief is experienced, felt, and expressed differently.

Each child goes through her own particular feelings at her own rate.

When my father died, I was stunned into silence. Someone else of my exact age might have launched into tears. And a third person might have escaped into a new romantic relationship.

Each child, each teenager, and for that matter, each adult who has lost a loved one needs and deserves to be treated as an individual with her own feelings and experience when she is grieving.

As you have read, loss in infancy and childhood affects that infant or child for the rest of her life.

And, as you have also read, the effect the loss has will be determined by the child's own personality, by her age, by the circumstances of the loss, by the child's life circumstances, and by the amount of help and support she receives following the loss.

It is for this reason that I have provided ways for you to understand what a child might be feeling given her age and stage of development, and ideas, tools, and guiding principles for how to help that child.

I sincerely hope that what you have read here will be of some help to you.

Corinne Masur

Chester Springs, Pennsylvania

March 2024

RESOURCES: BOOKS, PODCASTS, WEBSITES, AND MORE

Books for Adults

Notes on Grief, Chimamanda Ngozi Adichie

The Grieving Brain, Mary-Frances O'Connor

The Other Side of Sadness, George Bonanno

Ambiguous Loss: Learning to Live With Unresolved Grief, Pauline Boss

The Myth of Closure: Ambiguous Loss in a Time of Pandemic and Change, Pauline Boss

It's OK That You're Not OK: Meeting Grief and Loss in a Culture That Doesn't Understand, Megan Devine

Living When a Loved One Has Died, Earl Grollman

The Empty Room: Surviving the Loss of a Brother or Sister at Any Age, Elizabeth DeVita-Raeburn

Atlas of the Heart, Brené Brown

Bearing the Unbearable, Jeanne Cacciatore

The Year of Magical Thinking, Joan Didion

Resilient Grieving, Lucy Hone

Why Bad Things Happen to Good People, Harold Kushner

I Wasn't Ready to Say Goodbye, Brooke Noel

How to Go On When Someone You Love Dies, Therese A. Rando

Heartbroken: Healing From the Loss of a Spouse, Gary Roe

Helping Children Cope After a Traumatic Event: A Recovery Guide for Parents, Teachers and Community Leaders, Child Mind Institute

Books for Teachers and School Administrators

Helping the Grieving Student: A Guide for Teachers, the Dougy Center
When Death Impacts Your School: A Guide for School Administrators, the Dougy Center
Helping Children Cope After a Traumatic Event: A Recovery Guide for Parents, Teachers and Community Leaders, Child Mind Institute

Books for Parents

Children, Teens and Suicide Loss, the Dougy Center
Helping Children Cope with Death, the Dougy Center
Helping Teens Cope With Death, the Dougy Center
35 Ways to Help a Grieving Child, the Dougy Center
Never the Same: Coming to Terms With the Death of a Parent, Donna Shurman
Helping Children's Grief: Surviving a Parent's Death From Cancer, Grace Hyslop Christ

Books for Children

A Kid's Book About Grief, Brennan C. Wood. This book skillfully explains the mixture of emotions children can feel after a loss.
Grief Is a Mess, Jackie Shuld. Through humorous illustrations, this book explains how grief is different for everyone.
The Tenth Good Thing About Barney, Judith Viorst. A good beginning book about death, this one involves the death of a pet but treats the subject in a way that also explains the cycle of life.
Nana Upstairs, Nana Downstairs, Tomie dePaola. A gentle book about the death of a great-grandmother.
Memories Matter: 70 Activities for Grieving Children and Teens, the Dougy Center.
Lifetimes, the Beautiful Way to Explain Death to Children, Bryan Mellonie and Robert Ingpen. A sensitive book about beginnings and endings, especially for young children but suitable for people of all ages.
A Walk in the Woods, Nicki Grimes, Jerry Pinkney, and Brian Pinkney. A young boy goes on an adventure after his father's death.

Empty and Me, Azam Mahdavi. A little girl's experience with an imaginary friend after her mother dies.

Where Did Benjamin Go?, Chris Clarkson. A little boy named Charlie remembers his big brother who died.

Always Sisters, Saira Mir. A mother explains to her little girl that the baby sister they both looked forward to won't be coming home.

I Wish I Could Tell You, Jean-Francois Senechal. A little fox's grandmother dies.

Sylvester's Letter, Matthew Burgess. Letters can't be delivered in the usual way when they have to go all the way to Heaven.

Grief Is an Elephant, Tamara Ellis Smith. Grief starts out as an elephant and eventually shrinks to the size of a firefly.

Cape, Kevin Johnson. A little boy has to attend a funeral and puts on a big red cape to help him cope with the most painful of his feelings.

The Swing, Britta Tekentrup. For readers of all ages, these swings are both a place to fly and a place to be in quiet solitude.

The Bear and the Wildcat, Kazui Sakai. A bear mourns his bird friend.

My Friend Loonie, Nina La Cour. A little girl loses her balloon and learns that she can be sad for a while and then feel happy again.

Books for Teens

A Grieving Teen: A Guide for Teens and Friends, Helen Fitzgerald. A unique and compassionate guide in which grief counselor Helen Fitzgerald gives teens the tools they need to work through their pain and grief.

Straight Talk About Death for Teenagers: How to Cope with Losing Someone You Love, Earl A. Grollman. What to expect when you lose someone you love.

Podcasts for Adults

All There Is: A podcast about loss (for older teens and adults) by Anderson Cooper.

Good Mourning: Sally Douglas and Imogen Carn talk about loss and grief in a world where it seems to be taboo.

Dealing With My Grief: This podcast follows Darwyn M. Dave, who lost his father in 1978 when he was ten years old. As time went on, he realized he wasn't over it, and his grief was impacting his life in big ways. He started this podcast to share his coping mechanisms with others experiencing grief and loss.

End of Life University: Hospice physician and author Dr. Karen Wyatt outlines all that end-of-life care entails; burials, planning, and, of course, grief.

Grief and Guts: Melissa Dlugolecki discusses the tragic loss of a baby.

Griefcast: A podcast on grief through the lens of comedy.

The Grief Gang: Host Amber Jeffrey talks about the unexpected loss of her mother when she was nineteen.

Grief Is a Sneaky Bitch: Lisa Keefauver provides raw and honest discussions about grief and the conversations we can have about it.

Grief Out Loud: A podcast from the acclaimed Dougy Center, featuring children, teens, and adults sharing their stories.

The Grief Refuge: Reid Peterson provides conversations and helpful information about grief, loss, and managing the process. Filled with insights and creative ideas for navigating grief's difficult emotions, the Grief Refuge podcast educates, soothes, and comforts anyone who is trying to understand what they're going through.

The Grief Sofa: Stories of grief and mourning hosted by Alice Williams and Lucy Dennis. Join them for weekly episodes welcoming guests who share stories of those lost along the way. Find them on Instagram at @thegriefsofa or email thegriefsofa@gmail.com.

Grief Uncensored: This podcast, hosted by Julia Gallegos and Yako Shirasuna, was created to uncover the reality behind a heartbreaking tragedy: losing a parent way too soon. Both hosts lost a parent in their last semester of college.

Grief Unfiltered: Talking about grief when no one else seems to be talking about it. Hosted by Jayme Allis.

Mindfulness and Grief: For those who have lost someone recently as well as for professionals in the field of grief. Hosted by Heather Stang.

Terrible, Thanks for Asking: Nora McInerny lost her father, her husband, and her unborn child all within a year.

Unlocking US: Brené Brown on mental health and the conversations that we can have about grief and loneliness.

What's Your Grief?: This podcast provides resources, personal stories, and coping skills to those grieving. It comes from the mental health website of the same name and is hosted by mental health professionals Eleanor Haley and Litsa Williams. Topics include how to not avoid your grief and grief expectations.

Where's the Grief?: Hosted by comedian Jordan Ferber, this podcast includes stories of various kinds of loss and grief.

See this link for more: https://www.choosingtherapy.com/grief-podcasts/.

Online Support Groups

Grief in Common
   https://www.griefincommon.com
Grief Anonymous
   https://www.griefanonymous.com/
HealGrief: Actively Moving Forward
   https://healgrief.org/actively-moving-forward/
HEARTBEAT: Grief Support After Suicide
   https://www.heartbeatsurvivorsaftersuicide.org
Soaring Spirits International: Widowed Village
   https://soaringspirits.org
Widows and Widowers Grief Support Group
   https://nationalwidowers.org/support-groups/
   https://sisterhoodofwidows.com
Young Widows/Widowers Support Club (find on Facebook)
Compassionate Friends: For Those Who Have Lost a Child
   https://www.compassionatefriends.org
The Widowed Parent, University of North Carolina: A new online resource specifically for parents who have lost a spouse or partner and are raising children on their own.
   http://www.widowedparent.org/
Cancer Support Community, Benjamin Center
   https://www.cancersupportcommunity.org/

Therapy Resources

Psychology Today, https://www.psychologytoday.com/us

Other Resources for Children

Apart of Me: An in-app game for mobile devices that can be downloaded via App Store or Google Play (depending on the device's operational system). To find out how to access the game, go to the home page at https://www.apartofme.app/. To find out more about Apart of Me, go to https://www.apartofme.app/about.

The people who create Sesame Street have provided numerous wonderful resources for children regarding grief and loss: https://sesameworkshop .org/topics/grief/

Blogs for Adults

A Lovely Woman by Carmel Breathnach:
     www.alovelywoman.wordpress.com
What's Your Grief: Readers share and support one another.
     www.whatsyourgrief.com
Grief Healing: Useful information on caregiving, grief and transition for adults coping with loss.
     www.griefhealingblog.com
Modern Loss: Conversations about grief
     www.modernloss.com
Grief by Mark Liebenow: For widowers
     www.widowersgrief.blogspot.com
Widow's Voice: For widows
     www.widowsvoice.com
Art Therapy and Mental Health Blog
     www.arttherapyblog.com/c/mental-health/

Important Organizations

The Dougy Center, The National Grief Center for Children and Families: This center provides direct services to children and families in Portland,

Oregon, but it is also a clearinghouse for information on grief for people all over the US and the world. The Dougy Center sells a number of excellent publications on grief in childhood and adolescence through its bookstore, and it provides resources for professionals. Its website is devoted to finding grief support groups in your area. www.dougy.org

The Center for Loss and Bereavement: www.bereavementcenter.org/clb -grief-resources/

National Alliance for Children's Grief: www.nacg.org

The Grief Recovery Method: The Action Progra for Moving Beyond Loss: www.grief-recovery.com

Grief Camps for Children

Camp Erin: Children and teens ages 6–17 attend a weekend camp that combines traditional, fun camp activities with grief education and emotional support, free of charge for all families. Led by grief professionals and trained volunteers, Camp Erin is offered in every Major League Baseball city and other locations across the US. https:// elunanetwork.org/camps-programs/camp-erin/

Camp Courage: Camp Courage is for children ages 7–18 and allows campers to come together with other children and teens who have experienced similar losses as they learn new ways of dealing with their grief. The weekend camp has many fun activities and has a professional counselor, nurse, and volunteers. https://www.geisinger.org /patient-care/specialty/home-health-hospice/hhh-camp-courage

Comfort Zone Camp: Comfort Zone Camp includes confidence building programs and age-based support groups that break emotional isolation. Campers engage in resilience training programs while also having playing games, singing, and doing skits. Camps are available for children ages 7–17 and are offered across the country. https:// comfortzonecamp.org/calendar/

HOW TO HELP GRIEVING CHILDREN CHECKLIST

As you help your grieving child, feel free to refer back to this checklist for a reminder of the major ways you can be there during their time of mourning.

1. **Be available.** Spend time with the child, listen to the child, talk about your own feelings when you have experienced loss.

2. **Listen more, talk less.** Listen to what the child has to say and the questions the child has. Talk about your own feelings only if you think the child would like to hear from you or if you think she needs help figuring out how to feel and how to mourn.

3. **Be ready for questions.** Answer all questions no matter how difficult, keeping in mind the age and stage of development of the child asking. For younger children, use simple language and simple ideas. Be concrete. For older children, add more complexity to your answers.

4. **Bring in others to help.** Your child needs all the help she can get at this time. If your child gives you permission, tell her teacher about the loss and ask the teacher to be sensitive to the feelings your child may be having, which may affect her performance and/or behavior in school. Bring in others who love your child—aunts, uncles, grandparents, cousins, family friends, etc., to provide additional support.

5. **Respect the child's feelings.** If she prefers to spend some time alone, allow it. If she prefers to not talk about the loss for a few weeks, allow it.

6. **Don't be afraid to ask for professional help.** Seek a professional evaluation from a grief specialist, psychologist, or social worker if your child will not talk about the loss or prefers to spend time alone for more than a period of a few weeks to a month.

ACKNOWLEDGMENTS

Many thanks go to my agent, Jennifer Thompson, without whose faith in me, this book would never have gone to print. Thank you also to Laura Apperson, my editor, and to Rachel Ottman, my indefatigable research assistant. Particular thanks, of course, go to all the children and teens who have taught me about grief—and especially to Teigan, Lucine, and Henry from Winston's Wish, who talked to me about their private experiences of loss. I would also like to thank Terence Carroll for his patience, generosity, and affection, and TJ Fallon for his love and eternal tech support.

NOTES

Preface

1 William Shakespeare, *Folger Shakespeare Library* (New York: Simon & Schuster, 2003).

Introduction

1 Ariana Eunjung Cha, "10.5 Million Children Lost a Parent or Caregiver Because of Covid, Study Says," *Washington Post*, September 6, 2022, https://www.washingtonpost.com/health/2022/09/06/covid-deaths-orphans-worldwide/.

2 Susan Hillis et al., "Orphanhood and Caregiver Loss Among Children Based on New Global Excess COVID-19 Death Estimates," *JAMA Pediatrics* 176, no. 11 (November 2022): 1145–1148.

3 Lisa Berg, Mikael Rostila, and Anders Hjern, "Parental Death During Childhood and Depression in Young Adults—A National Cohort Study," *Journal of Child Psychology and Psychiatry* 57, no. 9 (September 2016): 1092–1098.

4 Benjamin Oosterhoff, Julie B. Kaplow, and Christopher M. Layne, "Links Between Bereavement Due to Sudden Death and Academic Functioning: Results from a Nationally Representative Sample of Adolescents," *School Psychology Quarterly* 33, no. 3 (September 2018): 372–380.

5 Mai-Britt Guldin et al., "Incidence of Suicide Among Persons Who Had a Parent Who Died During Their Childhood: A Population-Based Cohort Study," *JAMA Psychiatry* 72, no. 12 (December 2014): 1227–1234.

6 Michaeleen Burns et al., "Childhood Bereavement: Understanding Prevalence and Related Adversity in the United States," *American Journal of Orthopsychiatry* 90, no. 4 (2020): 391–405.

7 Elisabeth Kübler-Ross and David Kessler, *On Grief and Grieving: Finding the Meaning of Grief Through the Five Stages of Loss* (New York: Scribner, 2014).

Chapter 1

1   George A. Bonnano, "Loss, Trauma and Human Resilience: Have We Underestimated the Human Capacity to Thrive After Extremely Aversive Events?" *American Psychologist* 59, no. 1 (January 2004): 20–28.

2   M. W. deVries, "Temperament and Infant Mortality Among the Masai of East Africa," *American Journal of Psychiatry* 141, no. 10 (October 1984): 1189–1194, https://doi.org/10.1176/ajp.141.10.1189.

3   Ann S. Masten, "Global Perspectives on Resilience in Children and Youth," *Child Development* 85, no. 1 (December 2013): 6–20.

4   Séamas O'Reilly, *Did Ye Hear Mammy Died?* (New York: Little, Brown, 2021).

5   O'Reilly, *Did Ye Hear Mammy Died?*.

6   Geddam Subhasree et al., "Personality Traits and Resilience of People with Bereaved Experiences Due to COVID-19: Mediating Role of Self-Efficacy," *Illness, Crises, and Loss* (May 2023), https://doi.org/10.1177/10541373231177417.

7   Lawrence G. Calhoun and Richard G. Tedeschi, "The Foundations of Posttraumatic Growth: An Expanded Framework," in *Handbook of Posttraumatic Growth: Research and Practice*, ed. Calhoun and Tedeschi (New Jersey: Lawrence Erlbaum, 2006), 3–23.

8   Richard G. Tedeschi and Lawrence G. Calhoun, "Posttraumatic Growth: A New Perspective on Psychotraumatology," *Psychiatric Times* 21, no. 4 (April 1, 2004).

9   Jessica Koblenz, "Growing from Grief: Qualitative Experiences of Parental Loss," *Omega* 73, no. 3 (March 2015): 203–230.

10 Helen Macdonald, *H Is for Hawk* (New York: Grove Atlantic, 2015).

11 D. W. Winnicott, *The Piggle: An Account of the Psychanalytic Treatment of a Little Girl* (London: Penguin Books, 1977)

Chapter 2

1   Donald Winnicott, *The Maturational Process and the Facilitating Environment* (London: Routledge, 1990).

2   John Bowlby, *Attachment*, 2nd ed., vol. 1, Attachment and Loss Series (New York: Basic Books Classics, 1983).

3   Susan Coates, *Trauma and Human Bonds* (London: Routledge, 2016).

4   Coates, *Trauma and Human Bonds*.

5   Ian Bushnell, "Mother's Face Recognition in Newborn Infants: Learning and Memory," *Infant and Child Development* 10, no. 1–2 (2001): 67–74, https://doi.org/10.1002/icd.248.

6   M. Klaus and J. Kennel, *Mother-Infant Bonding* (St. Louis: E. V. Mosely, 1976).

7   Beatrice Beebe and Frank M. Lachman, *The Origins of Attachment: Infant Research and Adult Treatment* (London: Routledge, 2013).

8   Bowlby, *Attachment*; John Bowlby, *Separation: Anxiety and Anger*, vol. 2, Attachment and Loss Series (New York: Basic Books Classics, 1998); John Bowlby, *Loss: Sadness and Depression*, vol. 3, Attachment and Loss Series (New York: Basic Books Classics, 1998).

9   Harry Bakwin, "Loneliness in Infants," *American Journal of Diseases of Children* 63, no. 1 (January 1942): 30–40.

10   Bakwin, "Loneliness in Infants."

11   Donald Winnicott, John Bowlby, and Emanuel Miller, "Evacuation of Small Children," *British Medical Journal*, December 16, 1939.

12   D. Burlingham and A. Freud, *Young Children in War-time* (London: Allen and Unwin, 1942).

13   Frank C. P. van der Horst and Renée van der Veer, "The Ontogeny of an Idea: John Bowlby and Contemporaries on Mother-Child Separation," *History of Psychology* 13, no. 1 (February 2013): 25–45.

14   René A. Spitz, *The First Year of Life* (New York: International Universities Press, 1977).

15   Susan Coates, Jane Rosenthal, and Daniel Schechter, *September 11: Trauma and Human Bonds* (London: Routledge, 2003).

16   Margo S. Landers and Regina Sullivan, "The Development and Neurobiology of Infant Attachment and Fear," *Developmental Neuroscience* 34, no. 2–3 (2012): 101–114.

17   Gilbert Kliman, *Psychological Emergencies of Childhood* (New York: Grune and Stratton, 1968).

18   James Agee, *A Death in the Family* (New York: McDowell, Obolensky, 2009), 241.

19   John Bowlby, *Attachment*, vol. 1 (New York: Basic Books Classics, 1983).

20   Agee, *A Death in the Family*.

21   Agee, *A Death in the Family*.

22   Séamas O'Reilly, *Did Ye Hear Mammy Died?* (New York: Little, Brown, 2021)

Chapter 3

1   Erna Furman, *A Child's Parent Dies* (New Haven: Yale University Press, 1974).

2   Maxine Harris, *The Loss That Is Forever* (New York: Penguin, 1995).

3   James Agee, *A Death in the Family* (New York: McDowell, Obolensky, 2009), 306.

4   Agee, *A Death in the Family*.

5   Séamas O'Reilly, *Did Ye Hear Mammy Died?* (New York: Little, Brown, 2022).

6   Eliza Griswold, "The Kids Who Lost Parents to Covid," *New Yorker*, July 13, 2022.

7   O'Reilly, *Did Ye Hear Mammy Died?*

8   Elizabeth DeVita-Raeburn, *The Empty Room: Understanding Sibling Loss* (New York: Scribner, 2007), 21–22.

9   DeVita-Raeburn, *The Empty Room*.

Chapter 4

1   Grace Hyslop Christ, *Helping the Grieving Child* (Oxford: Oxford University Press, 2000).

2   Christ, *Helping the Grieving Child*.

3   Christ, *Helping the Grieving Child*.

4   Christ, *Helping the Grieving Child*.

5   Education Week, Jan. 6, 2023, "School Sshootings this Yyear: Hhow Mmany and Wwhere,." *Education Week*, January 6, 2023, https://www.edweek.org /leadership/school-shootings-this-year-how-many-and-where/2023/01.

6   CNN Staff, "Florida Student Emma Gonzalez to Lawmakers and Gun Advocates: 'We Call BS,'" CNN, February 17, 2018, https://www.cnn.com/2018/02 /17/us/florida-student-emma-gonzalez-speech/.

7   "Parkland Survivor Eden Hebron Credits Intervention With Saving Her Life," CBS News, Miami, May 7, 2022.

8   Eli Saslo, "When Back to School Means Reliving the Worst Day in Your Life," *New York Times*, September 29, 2023.

9   Gudrun Østby, Siri Aas Rustad, and Andreas Forø Tollefsen, "Children Affected by Armed Conflict, 1990–2019," *Conflict Trends* 6.

10 Theresa S. Betancourt et al., "The Intergenerational Impact of War on Mental Health and Psychosocial Wellbeing: Lessons from the Longitudinal Study of War-Affected Youth in Sierra Leone," *Conflict and Health* 14, no. 62 (2020), https://doi.org/10.1186/s13031-020-00308-7.

11 United Nations High Commission on Refugees Global Report, Geneva, Switzerland, 2022, https://reporting.unhcr.org/global-report-2022.

12 Christina W. Hoven et al., "Parental Exposure to Mass Violence and Child Mental Health: The First Responder and WTC Evacuee Study," *Clinical Child and Family Psychology Review* 12, no. 2 (June 2009): 95–112.

13 Mona El-Naggar, Jonah M. Kessel, and Alexander Stockton, "What Is War to a Grieving Child?" *New York Times*, July 18, 2023.

14 David Bürgin et al., "Impact of War and Forced Displacement on Children's Mental Health—Multilevel, Needs-Oriented, and Trauma-Informed Approaches," *European Child & Adolescent Psychiatry* 31, no. 6 (June 2022): 845–853, https://doi.org/10.1007/s00787-022-01974-z.

15 Vathsalan Sriskandarajah, Frank Neuner, and Claudia Catani, "Parental Care Protects Traumatized Sri Lankan Children from Internalizing Behavior Problems," *BMC Psychiatry* 15 (2015).

16 Regina Saile et al., "Children of the Postwar Years: A Two-Generational Multilevel Risk Assessment of Child Psychopathology," *Development and Psychopathology* 28, no. 2 (May 2016): 607–662.

17 Anna Freud and Dorothy T. Burlingham, *War and Children* (New York: Medical War Books, 1943).

18 Francesco Bisagni, "Shrapnel: Latency, Mourning and the Suicide of a Parent," *Journal of Child Psychotherapy* 38, no. 1 (March 2012): 22–31.

19 Julie Cerel and Timothy A. Roberts, "Suicidal Behavior in the Family and Adolescent Risk Behavior," *Journal of Adolescent Health* 36, no. 4 (April 2005): e9–e16.

Chapter 5

1 Pauline Boss, *Ambiguous Loss: Learning to Live with Unresolved Grief* (Cambridge, MA: Harvard University Press, 1999), 3.

2 Boss, *Ambiguous Loss*, 11.

3 Kenneth J. Doka, *Disenfranchised grief: Recognizing hidden sorrow* (Maryland: Lexington Books/D. C. Heath and Com, 1989), xv.

4   Pauline Boss, *The Myth of Closure: Ambiguous Loss in a Time of Pandemic and Change* (New York: Norton, 2022).

5   Teresa Pham-Carsillo, "My (Liberating) Secret Shame," *New York Times*, October 8, 2023.

6   Boss, *Ambiguous Loss*, 5.

7   Boss, *Ambiguous Loss*, 6.

8   Julie Kim, "Grieving the Future I Imagined for My Daughter," *The Atlantic*, April 22, 2019, https://www.theatlantic.com/family/archive/2019/04/1p36 -genetic-disorder-reshaping-my-family/586717/.

Chapter 7

1   Donna L. Schuurman, *Helping Children Cope with Death* (Portland, OR: Dougy Center, 1998).

2   Schuurman, *Helping Children Cope with Death*.

3   Schuurman, *Helping Children Cope with Death*.

4   Grace Hyslop Christ, *Healing Children's Grief* (Oxford: Oxford University Press, 2000).

5   Christ, *Healing Children's Grief*.

6   Christ, *Healing Children's Grief*.

7   Christ, *Healing Children's Grief*.

8   Christ, *Healing Children's Grief*.

9   Christ, *Healing Children's Grief*.

10   Schuurman, *Helping Children Cope with Death*.

11   Schuurman, *Helping Children Cope with Death*.

12   D. Glicken, "The Child's View of Death," *Journal of Marital and Family Therapy* 4, no. 2 (1978): 75–81.

13   Carmel Breathnach, "My Burning Desire to Write 'Briefly I Knew My Mother,'" *A Lovely Woman*, WordPress Blog, May 17, 2016.

14   Christ, *Healing Children's Grief*.

Chapter 8

1   *Helping Children Cope with Death*, the Dougy Center, National Center for Grieving Children and Families, Portland, OR, 2004.

2   Grace Hyslop Christ, *Healing Children's Grief* (Oxford: Oxford University Press, 2000), 147.

3   Elizabeth DeVita-Raeburn, *The Empty Room: Understanding Sibling Loss* (New York: Scribner, 2007).

4   AACAP, "Video Games and Children: Playing with Violence," *American Academy of Child and Adolescent Psychiatry* 91 (June 2017), https://www.aacap.org/AACAP/Families_and_Youth/Facts_for_Families/FFF-Guide/Children-and-Video-Games-Playing-with-Violence-091.aspx.

5   https://nhttac.acf.hhs.gov/soar/eguide/stop/adverse_childhood_experiences.

6   Julie Kaplow, "Helping Kids Cope with Trauma and Grief Related to Gun Violence," Childrens' Hospital New Orleans, August 30, 2022, https://chnola.org/news-blog/2022/august/helping-kids-cope-with-trauma-and-grief-related-/.

7   Kaplow, "Helping Kids Cope with Trauma and Grief."

8   Kaplow, "Helping Kids Cope with Trauma and Grief."

9   Kaplow, "Helping Kids Cope with Trauma and Grief."

Chapter 9

1   Paul M. Brinich, "Death and the Schools: A Psychological Plan of Action," *Psychoanalytic Study of the Child* 72, no. 1 (April 2019): 228–240.

2   Kiese Layman, "In 'Memorial Drive' a Poet Evokes Her Childhood and Confronts Her Mother's Murder," *New York Times*, July 30, 2020, https://www.nytimes.com/2020/07/30/books/review/memorial-drive-natastha-trethewey.html.

3   Jessica Koblenz, "Growing from Grief: Qualitative Experiences of Parental Loss," *Omega* 73, no. 3 (March 2015).

4   Alan Carr, *What Works with Children and Adolescents? A Critical Review of Psychological Interventions with Children, Adolescents, and Their Families* (London: Routledge, 2000).

5   Susan Coates, *September 11: Trauma and Human Bonds* (London: Routledge, 2003).

6   Personal communication, 1984.

7   Coates, *September 11*, 46.

8   Coates, *September 11*.

9   Thomas Lopez and Gilbert W. Kliman, "Memory, Reconstruction, and Mourning in the Analysis of a Four-Year-Old Child," *Psychoanalytic Study of the Child* 34, no. 1 (1979): 235–271.

10 Yvon Gauthier, "The Mourning Reaction of a Ten-Year-Old Boy," *Canadian Psychiatric Association Journal* 11 (1966): 487.

11 Lopez and Kliman, "Memory, Reconstruction, and Mourning," 266.

12 Mariken Spuij, Annemarie van Londen-Huiberts, and Paul A. Boelen, "Cognitive-Behavioral Therapy for Prolonged Grief in Children: Feasibility and Multiple Baseline Study," *Cognitive and Behavioral Practice* 20, no. 3 (August 2013): 349–361.

13 Paul A. Boelen, Lonneke I. M. Lenferink, and Mariken Spuij, "CBT for Prolonged Grief in Children and Adolescents: A Randomized Clinical Trial," *American Journal of Psychiatry* 178, no. 4 (January 2021): 294–304, https://doi.org/10.1176/appi.ajp.2020.20050548.

14 Perihan Aral Rosenthal, "Short-Term Family Therapy and Pathological Grief Reactions with Children and Adolescents," *Family Process* 19, no. 2 (June 1980): 151–159.

15 Jessica Koblenz, "Growing from Grief: Qualitative Experience of Parental Loss," *Omega* 73, no. 3 (March 2015): 203–230.

16 Jillian M. Blueford, Nancy E. Thacker, and Pamelia E. Bott, "Creating a System of Care for Early Adolescents Grieving a Death-Related Loss," *Journal of Child and Adolescent Counseling* 7, no. 3 (November 2021): 207–220.

17 Blueford, Thacker, and Bott, "Creating a System of Care for Early Adolescents."

Chapter 10

1   Paul A. Boelen et al., "Prolonged Grief and Depression After Unnatural Loss," *Psychiatry Research* 240 (June 2016): 358–363.

2   Natasha Trethewey, *Memorial Drive* (New York: Ecco, 2020), 205.

3   Bessel van der Kolk, *The Body Keeps the Score: Brain, Mind and Body in the Healing of Trauma* (New York: Penguin, 2014)

4   Vivien Dent, "When the Body Keeps the Score," *Psychoanalytic Inquiry* 40, no. 6 (August 17, 2020), https://www.semanticscholar.org/paper/When-the-Body-Keeps-the-Score%3A-Some-Implications-of-Dent/3ceba399258c50713f41918e734794b36fb582af.

5   Susan Coates, *September 11: Trauma and Human Bonds* (London: Routledge, 2003).

6   Coates, *September 11.*

7   Áine Travers, Tracey McDonagh, and Ask Elklit, "Youth Responses to School Shootings: A Review," *Current Psychiatry Reports* 20 (2018): 47, https://doi .org/10.1007/s11920-018-0903-1.

8   American Psychiatric Association, "What Is Posttraumatic Stress Disorder (PTSD)?" https://www.psychiatry.org/patients-families/ptsd/what-is-ptsd.

9   Cindy Tofthagen et al., "Complicated Grief with Post-Traumatic Stress Disorder Addressed with Accelerated Resolution Therapy: Case Discussions," *Omega (Westport)* 85, no. 2 (June 2022): 455–464.

10 P. A. Johnson and P. C. Rosenblatt, "Grief Following Loss of a Parent," *American Journal of Psychotherapy* 35, no. 3 (July 1981): 419–425.

11 Johnson and Rosenblatt, "Grief Following Loss of a Parent."

Chapter 11

1   Séamas O'Reilly, *Did Ye Hear Mammy Died?* (New York: Little, Brown, 2021).

2   Natasha Trethewey, *Memorial Drive* (New York: Ecco, 2020), 205.

3   O'Reilly, *Did Ye Hear Mammy Died?*

4   O'Reilly, *Did Ye Hear Mammy Died?*

5   O'Reilly, *Did Ye Hear Mammy Died?*

6   Sigmund Freud, *Mourning and Melancholia* (London: Hogarth, 1917), 237–258.

7   Pauline Boss, *The Myth of Closure: Ambiguous Loss in a Time of Pandemic and Change* (New York: Norton, 2021), xvi.

8   Lawrence G. Calhoun and Richard G. Tedeschi, *Handbook of Posttraumatic Growth: Research and Practice* (London: Routledge, 2014).

9   Todd B. Kashdan and Jennifer Q. Kane, "Post-Traumatic Distress and the Presence of Post-Traumatic Growth and Meaning in Life: Experiential Avoidance as a Moderator," *Personality and Individual Differences* 50, no. 1 (January 2011): 84–89, https://doi.org/10.1016/j.paid.2010.08.028.

10 Jessica Koblenz, "Growing from Grief: Qualitative Experiences of Parental Loss," *Omega* 73, no. 3 (2016): 203–230.

BIBLIOGRAPHY

Agee, James. *A Death in the Family.* New York: McDowell, Obolensky, 1957.

AACAP. "Video Games and Children: Playing with Violence." *American Academy of Child and Adolescent Psychiatry* 91 (June 2017).

American Psychiatric Association (APA). "What Is Post Traumatic Stress Disorder (PTSD)?" https://www.psychiatry.org/patients-families/ptsd/what-is-ptsd.

Bakwin, Harry. "Loneliness in Infants." *American Journal of Diseases of Children* 63, no. 1 (January 1942): 30–40.

Beebe, Beatrice, and Frank M. Lachman. *The Origins of Attachment: Infant Research and Adult Treatment.* London: Routledge, 2013.

Berg, Lisa, Mikael Rostila, and Anders Hjern. "Parental Death During Childhood and Depression in Young Adults—A National Cohort Study." *Journal of Child Psychology and Psychiatry* 57, no. 9 (September 2016): 1092–1098.

Betancourt, Theresa S., Katrina Keegan, Jordan Farrar, and Robert T. Brennan. "The Intergenerational Impact of War on Mental Health and Psychosocial Wellbeing: Lessons from the Longitudinal Study of War-Affected Youth in Sierra Leone." *Conflict and Health* 14, no. 62 (2020). https://doi.org/10.1186/s13031-020-00308-7.

Bisagni, Francesco. "Shrapnel: Latency, Mourning and the Suicide of a Parent." *Journal of Child Psychotherapy* 38, no. 1 (March 2012): 22–31.

Blueford, Jillian M., Nancy E. Thacker, and Pamelia E. Bott. "Creating a System of Care for Early Adolescents Grieving a Death-Related Loss." *Journal of Child and Adolescent Counseling* 7, no. 3 (November 2021): 1–14. https://doi.org/10.1080/23727810.2021.1973262.

Bonnano, George. "Loss, Trauma and Human Resilience: Have We Underestimated the Human Capacity to Thrive After Extremely Aversive Events?" *American Psychologist* 59, no. 1 (January 2004): 20–28.

Boelen, Paul A., Lonneke I. M. Lenferink, and Mariken Spuij. "CBT for Prolonged Grief in Children and Adolescents: A Randomized Clinical Trial." *American*

Journal of Psychiatry 178, no. 4 (April 2021): 294–304. https://doi.org/10.1176 /appi.ajp.2020.20050548.

Boelen, Paul A., Albert Reijntjes, A. A. A. Manik J. Djelantik, and Geert E. Smid. "Prolonged Grief and Depression After Unnatural Loss: Latent Class Analyses and Cognitive Correlates." *Psychiatry Research* 240 (June 2016): 358–363.

Boss, Pauline. *Ambiguous Loss: Learning to Live with Unresolved Grief.* London: Harvard University Press, 2000.

———. *The Myth of Closure: Ambiguous Loss in a Time of Pandemic and Change.* New York: Norton, 2022.

Bowlby, John. *Attachment.* 2nd ed., vol. 1. Attachment and Loss Series. New York: Basic Books Classics, 1983.

———. *Attachment: Separation and Loss.* Vol. 2. New York: Basic Books Classics, 1976.

———. *Loss: Sadness and Depression.* Vol. 3. Attachment and Loss Series. New York: Basic Books Classics, 1998.

Breathnach, Carmel. "My Burning Desire to Write 'Briefly I Knew My Mother.'" *A Lovely Woman* (blog), May 17, 2016.

Brinich, Paul M. "Death and the Schools: A Psychological Plan of Action." *Psychoanalytic Study of the Child* 72, no. 1 (April 2019): 228–240.

Bürgin, David, Dimitris Anagnostopoulos, Board and Policy Division of ESCAP, Benedetto Vitiello, Thorsten Sukale, Marc Schmid, and Jörg M. Fegert. "Impact of War and Forced Displacement on Children's Mental Health—Multilevel, Needs-Oriented, and Trauma-Informed Approaches." *European Child and Adolescent Psychiatry* 31, no. 6 (June 2022): 845–853. https://doi .org/10.1007/s00787-022-01974-z.

Burlingham, Dorothy, and Anna Freud. *Young Children in Wartime.* London: Allen and Unwin, 1942.

Burns, Michaeleen, Brook Griese, Samuel King, and Ayelet Talmi. "Childhood Bereavement: Understanding Prevalence and Related Adversity in the United States." *American Journal of Orthopsychiatry* 90, no. 4 (January 2020): 391–405.

Bushnell, Ian W. R. "Mother's Face Recognition in Newborn Infants: Learning and Memory." *Infant and Child Development* 10, no. 1–2 (March 2001): 67–74.

Calhoun, Lawrence G., and Richard G. Tedeschi. "The Foundations of Posttraumatic Growth: An Expanded Framework." In *Handbook of Posttraumatic Growth: Research and Practice*, edited by Calhoun and Tedeschi, 3–23. New Jersey: Lawrence Erlbaum, 2006.

Calhoun, Lawrence G., and Richard G. Tedeschi, eds. *Handbook of Posttraumatic Growth: Research and Practice*. London: Routledge, 2014.

Carr, Alan. *What Works with Children and Adolescents? A Critical Review of Psychological Interventions with Children, Adolescents, and Their Families*. Florence, KY: Taylor and Francis, 2000.

Cerel, Julie, and Timothy A. Roberts. "Suicidal Behavior in the Family and Adolescent Risk Behavior." *Journal of Adolescent Health* 36, no. 4 (April 2005): 316–359.

Cha, Ariana E. "10.5 Million Children Lost a Parent or Caregiver Because of Covid, Study Says." *Washington Post*, September 6, 2022.

Christ, Grace Hyslop. *Helping the Grieving Child*. Oxford: Oxford University Press, 2000.

CNN Staff. "Florida Student Emma Gonzalez to Lawmakers and Gun Advocates: 'We call BS.'" CNN, February 17, 2018. https://www.cnn.com/2018/02/17/us/florida-student-emma-gonzalez-speech/.

Coates, Susan, Jane Rosenthal, and Daniel Schechter. *Trauma and Human Bonds*. London: Routledge, 2003.

Dent, Vivien. "When the Body Keeps the Score: Some Implications of Trauma Theory and Practice for Psychoanalytic Work." *Psychoanalytic Inquiry* 40, no. 6 (August 2020): 435–447.

DeVita-Raeburn, Elizabeth. *The Empty Room: Understanding Sibling Loss*. New York: Scribner, 2007.

deVries, M. W. "Temperament and Infant Mortality Among the Masai of East Africa." *American Journal of Psychiatry* 141, no. 10 (October 1984): 1189–1194.

Education Week. "School Shootings This Year: How Many and Where." *Education Week*, January 6, 2023.

El-Naggar, Mona, Jonah M. Kessel, and Alexander Stockton. "What Is War to a Grieving Child?" *New York Times*, July 18, 2023. https://www.nytimes.com/2023/07/18/opinion/ukraine-russia-war-children.html.

Freud, Sigmund. *Mourning and Melancholia*. London: Hogarth, 1917.

Furman, Erna. *A Child's Parent Dies*. New Haven, CT: Yale University Press, 1974.

Gauthier, Yvon. "The Mourning Reaction of a Ten-Year-Old Boy." *Canadian Psychiatric Association Journal* 11 (1966): 307–308.

Griswold, Eliza. "The Kids Who Lost Parents to Covid." *New Yorker*, July 13, 2022.

Guldin, Mai-Britt, Jiong Li, Henrik S. Pedersen, Carsten Obel, Esben Agerbo, Mika Gissler, Sven Cnattingius, Jørn Olsen, and Mogens Vestergaard. "Incidence of Suicide Among Persons Who Had a Parent Who Died During Their Childhood: A Population-Based Cohort Study." *JAMA Psychiatry* 72, no. 12 (December 2015): 1227–1234.

Harris, Maxine. *The Loss That Is Forever.* New York: Penguin, 1995.

Hill, Ryan M., Benjamin Oosterhoff, Christopher M. Layne, Evan Rooney, Stephanie Yudovich, Robert S. Pynoos, and Julie B. Kaplow. "Multidimensional Grief Therapy: Pilot Open Trail of a Novel Intervention for Bereaved Children and Adolescents." *Journal of Child and Family Studies* 28 (June 2019): 3062–3074. https://doi.org/10.1007/s10826-019-01481-x.

Hillis, Susan, Joel-Pascal Ntwali N'konzi, William Msemburi, Lucie Cluver, Andrés Villaveces, Seth Flaxman, and H. Juliette T. Unwin. "Orphanhood and Caregiver Loss Among Children Based on New Global Excess COVID-19 Death Estimates." *JAMA Pediatrics* 176, no. 11 (September 2022): 1145–1148.

Hoven, Christina W., Christiane S. Duarte, Ping Wu, Thao Doan, Navya Singh, Donald J. Mandell, Fan Bin, Yona Teichman, Meir Teichman, Judith Wicks, George Musa, and Patricia Cohen. "Parental Exposure to Mass Violence and Child Mental Health: The First Responder and WTC Evacuee Study." *Clinical Child and Family Psychology Review* 12, no. 2 (June 2009): 95–112.

Johnson, P. A., and P. C. Rosenblatt. "Grief Following Childhood Loss of a Parent." *American Journal of Psychotherapy* 35, no. 3 (July 1981): 419–425.

Kaplow, Julie. "Helping Kids Cope with Trauma and Grief Related to Gun Violence." Children's Hospital New Orleans, August 30, 2022. https://www .chnola.org/news-blog/2022/august/helping-kids-cope-with-trauma-and -grief-related-/.

Kashdan, Todd B., and Jennifer Q. Kane. "Post-Traumatic Distress and the Presence of Post-Traumatic Growth and Meaning in Life: Experiential Avoidance as a Moderator." *Personality and Individual Differences* 50, no. 1 (January 2011): 84–89. https://doi.org/10.1016/j.paid.2010.08.028.

Kaufman, Scott Barry. "Post-Traumatic Growth: Finding Meaning and Creativity in Adversity." *Scientific American*, April 20, 2020.

Kim, Julie. "Grieving the Future I Imagined for My Daughter." *The Atlantic*, April 22, 2019. https://www.theatlantic.com/family/archive/2019/04/1p36 -genetic-disorder-reshaping-my-family/586717/.

Klaus, Marshall H., and John H. Kennel. *Mother-Infant Bonding*. St. Louis: Mosely, 1976.

Kliman, Gilbert W. (1968). *Psychological Emergencies of Childhood*. New York: Grune and Stratton, 1968.

Koblenz, Jessica. "Growing from Grief: Qualitative Experiences of Parental Loss." *Omega* 73, no. 3 (March 2015): 203–230.

Kübler-Ross, Elisabeth, and David Kessler. *On Grief and Grieving: Finding the Meaning of Grief Through the Five Stages of Loss*. New York: Scribner, 2014.

Landers, Margo S., and Regina M. Sullivan. "The Development and Neurobiology of Infant Attachment and Fear." *Developmental Neuroscience* 34, no. 2–3 (May 2012): 101–114.

Layman, Kiese M. "In 'Memorial Drive' a Poet Evokes Her Childhood and Confronts Her Mother's Murder." *New York Times*, July 30, 2020.

Liu, M. "War and Children." *American Journal of Psychiatry* 12, no. 7 (July 2017): 3–5. https://doi.org/10.1176/appi.ajp-rj.2017.120702.

Lopez, Thomas, and Gilbert W. Kliman. "Memory, Reconstruction, and Mourning in the Analysis of a Four-Year-Old Child." *Psychoanalytic Study of the Child* 34, no. 1 (1979): 235–271.

Masten, Ann S. "Global Perspectives on Resilience in Children and Youth." *Child Development* 85, no. 1 (December 2013): 6–20.

Macdonald, Helen. *H Is for Hawk*. New York: Grove Atlantic, 2015.

Oosterhoff, Benjamin, Julie B. Kaplow, and Christopher M. Layne. "Links Between Bereavement Due to Sudden Death and Academic Functioning: Results from a Nationally Representative Sample of Adolescents." *School Psychology Quarterly* 33, no. 3 (September 2018): 372–380.

O'Reilly, Séamas. *Did Ye Hear Mammy Died?* New York: Little, Brown, 2021.

Østby, Gudrun, Siri Aas Rustad, and Andreas F. Tollefsen. "Children Affected by Armed Conflict, 1990–2019." *Conflict Trends* 6 (2020).

Pham-Carsillo, Teresa. "My (Liberating) Secret Shame." *New York Times*, October 8, 2023.

Rosenthal, Perihan A. "Short-Term Family Therapy and Pathological Grief Reactions with Children and Adolescents." *Family Process* 19, no. 2 (June 1980): 151–159.

Saile, Regina, Verena Ertl, Frank Neuner, and Claudia Catani. "Children of the Postwar Years: A Two-Generational Multilevel Risk Assessment of Child Psychopathology." *Development and Psychopathology* 28, no. 2 (May 2016): 607–620.

Santa Barbara, Joanna. "Impact of War on Children and Imperative to End War." *Croatian Medical Journal* 47, no. 6 (December 2006): 891–894.

Saslow, Eli. "When Back to School Means Reliving the Worst Day in Your Life." *New York Times*, September 29, 2023.

Schuurman, Donna L. *Helping Children Cope with Death*. Portland, OR: Dougy Center, 1998.

Shakespeare, William. *Macbeth*. Folger Shakespeare Library, 2003.

Spitz, René A. *The First Year of Life*. New York: International Universities Press, 1977.

Spuij, Mariken, Annemarie van Londen-Huiberts, and Paul A. Boelen. "Cognitive-Behavioral Therapy for Prolonged Grief in Children: Feasibility and Multiple Baseline Study." *Cognitive and Behavioral Practice* 20, no. 3 (August 2013): 349–361.

Sriskandarajah, Vathsalan, Frank Neuner, and Claudia Catani. "Parental Care Protects Traumatized Sri Lankan Children from Internalizing Behavior Problems." *BMC Psychiatry* 15 (August 2015): 203.

Subhasree, Geddam, Jojo C. Eapen, Sundaramoorthy Jeyavel, and Deepthi D. P. "Personality Traits and Resilience of People with Bereaved Experiences Due to COVID-19." *Illness, Crisis & Loss*, May 29, 2023.

Tedeschi, Richard G., and Lawrence Calhoun. "Posttraumatic Growth: A New Perspective on Psychotraumatology." *Psychiatric Times* 21, no. 4 (April 2004).

Tofthagen, Cindy, Diego F. Hernandez, Tina M. Mason, Harleah G. Buck, and Kevin E. Kip. "Complicated Grief with Post-Traumatic Stress Disorder Addressed with Accelerated Resolution Therapy: Case Discussions." *Omega* 85, no. 2 (June 2022): 455–464.

Travers, Áine, Tracey McDonagh, and Ask Elklit. "Youth Responses to School Shootings: A Review." *Current Psychiatry Reports* 20 (May 2018): 47. https://doi.org/10.1007/s11920-018-0903-1.

United Nations High Commission on Refugees. Global Report. UNHCR, 2022.

Van der Kolk, Bessell. *The Body Keeps the Score: Brain, Mind and Body in the Healing of Trauma*. London, Penguin, 2014.

van der Horst, Frank C. P., and Renée van der Veer. "The Ontogeny of an Idea: John Bowlby and Contemporaries on Mother-Child Separation." *History of Psychology* 13, no. 1 (February 2010): 25–45.

Winnicott, Donald. *The Maturational Process and the Facilitating Environment*. London: Routledge, 1990.

————. *The Piggle: An Account of the Psychoanalytic Treatment of a Little Girl.* London: Penguin, 1977.

————. "Winnicott, Bowlby and Miller Publish Open Letter Warning Against Psychological Effects on Evacuated Children." Institute of Psychoanalysis, March 3, 1939. https://psychoanalysis.org.uk/who-we-are/100-years-of-history /winnicott-bowlby-and-miller-publish-open-letter-warning-against.

INDEX